KICK YOUR WAY TO

FITNESS

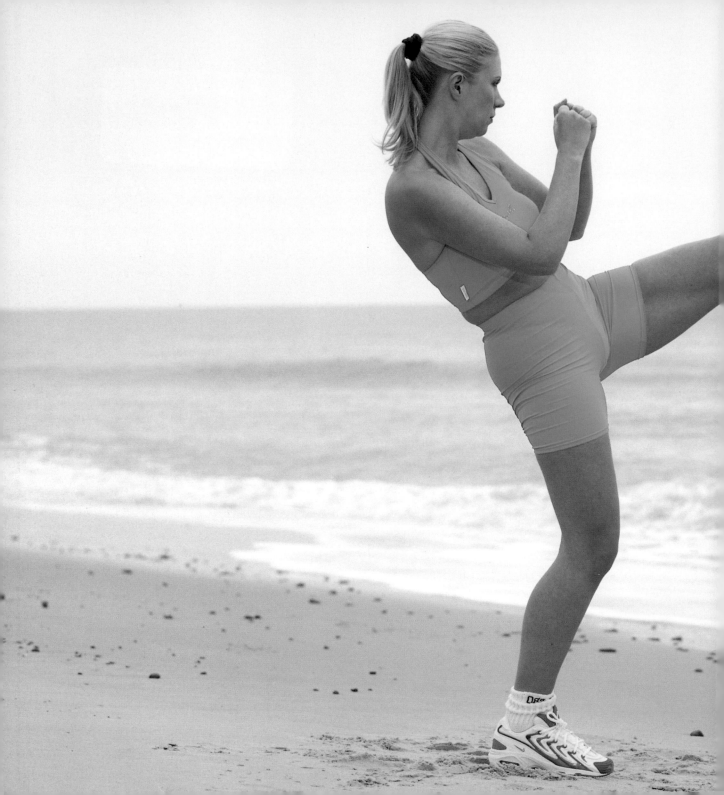

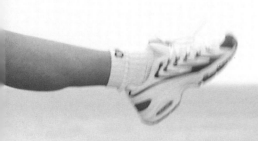

KICK YOUR WAY TO

FITNESS

**ANNE-MARIE MILLARD
AND SALLY BROWN**

Thorsons

Thorsons
An Imprint of HarperCollins*Publishers*
77–85 Fulham Palace Road
Hammersmith, London W6 8JB

The Thorsons website address is: www.thorsons.com

First published 2001

10 9 8 7 6 5 4 3 2 1

Text Copyright © Anne-Marie Millard and Sally Brown 2001
Copyright © HarperCollins*Publishers* Ltd 2001

Anne-Marie Millard and Sally Brown assert the moral right
to be identified as the authors of this work

Photographs by Robin Mathews

A catalogue record for this book is
available from the British Library

ISBN 0 00 710717 X

Printed and bound in Singapore for Imago

CONTENTS

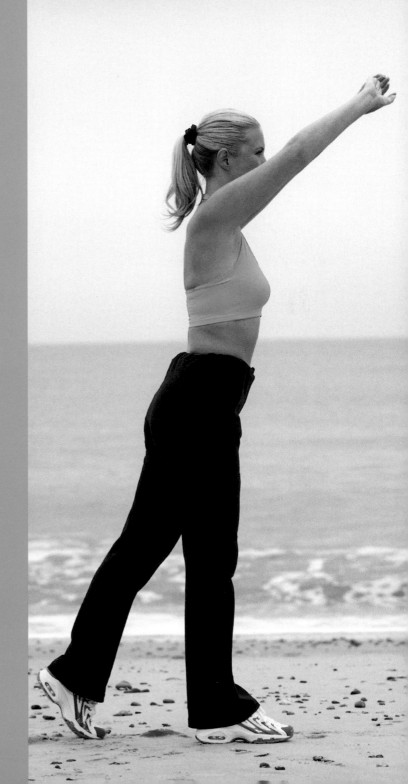

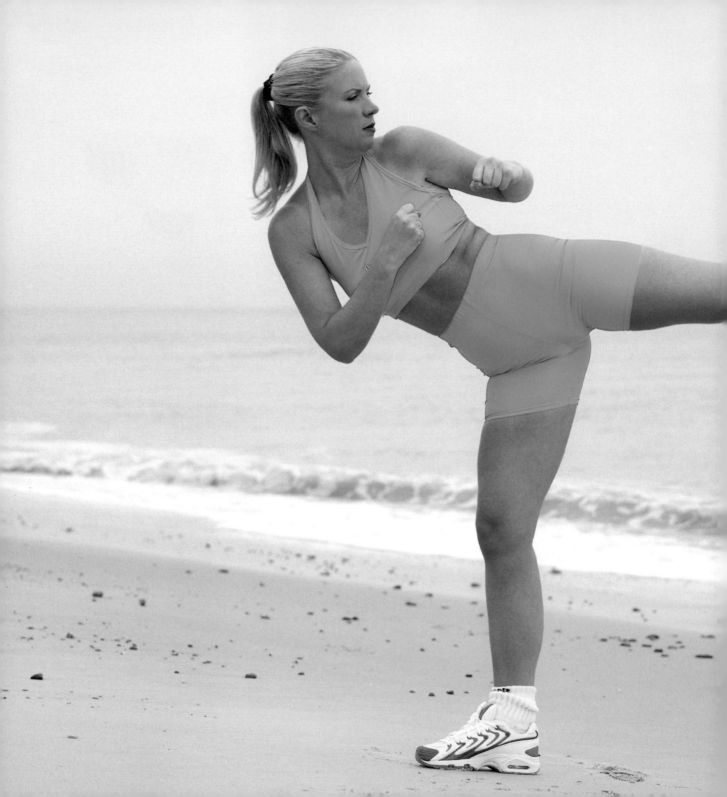

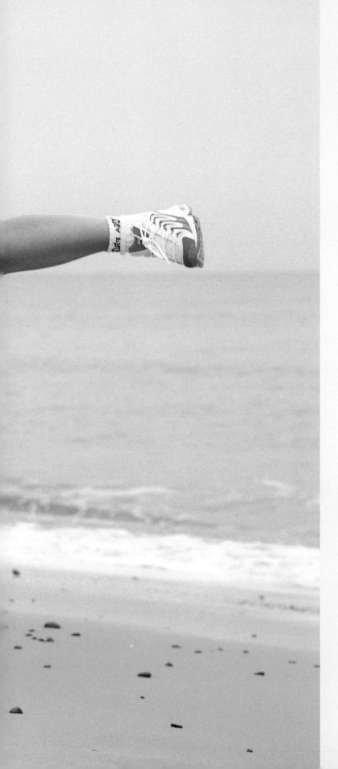

CHAPTER ONE

WHY KICK-IT! IS THE FUTURE OF FITNESS

How many of the following statements can you say 'yes' to?

- Every time I look in the mirror I feel unhappy at the sight of some part of my body.
- I try not to let my partner see me naked.
- I hate clothes shopping and end up buying what fits me or covers me up rather than what I really want.
- I have tried countless diets but I can never stick to them.
- I try to exercise but find going to the gym boring.
- I don't seem to eat more than most people and yet I'm always putting on weight.
- I have phases when I virtually starve myself, but then give up and end up eating more than ever.
- My friends and partner are sick of hearing me complaining about my weight.

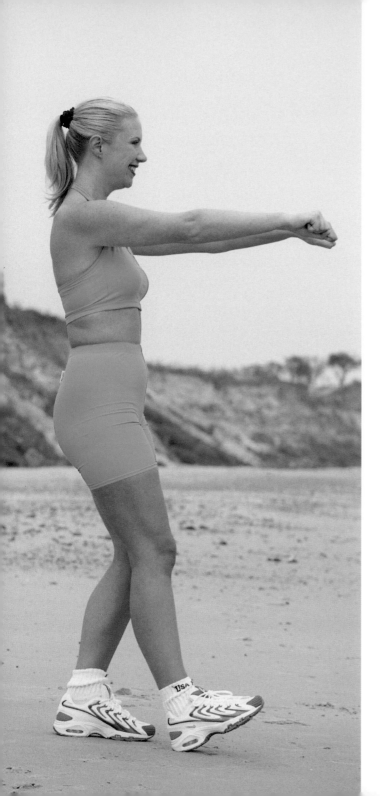

How do I know that you have experienced the things above? Because I have too, until the day that I met a Tae kwon do instructor and discovered that it is possible to have a sleek, lean body without dieting and while having fun. I now eat what I want and I'm a size 10. My secret is the style of training that I am about to describe in the chapters of this book. And the best part of all is that it is easy and enjoyable – believe me!

I was working in a gym and qualifying to be a fitness instructor when one day, I met Tessa. She was working out in the gym and had the most amazing body. I asked what she did to look like that. She told me she did Tae kwon do – a Korean-based martial art that involves lots of kicking moves – and that she taught at her own club (I later found out that she was also a world champion!). She told me to come along and try a class, but it took me another six months before I plucked up the courage.

I loved the atmosphere in the class, with the emphasis on respect for the teacher and senior class members, and personal humility. The class members came from all walks of life, egos were left at the gym door and respect had to be earned with diligence and hard work. I also liked the mental focus and concentration it required to get the moves right – it left no room for any other thoughts so I really blocked out everything else for the duration of the class, which was very liberating.

I was by no means a natural at it – in fact, my muscles had to learn to do the exact opposite of what I had been telling them to do after a childhood spent riding horses – i.e. to direct their power outwards, instead of inwards. But I persevered and was enjoying it so much that I hardly realized that it was also changing my body shape. I was becoming long and lean for the first time in my life.

It was a huge breakthrough for me because I had struggled with my weight all of my life. I grew up in a family where food was a central point of living and we had four substantial meals a day: breakfast, lunch, tea and dinner. So it's no surprise, really, that I was a plump child. At the same time, I was naturally sporty and active and rode horses from the age of four, so as well as being well-built, I was solid and muscular – I looked like a little boxer.

It didn't really bother me until I was about 16 and that's when it started going wrong. It's a familiar tale. First I started trying to control my weight by not eating but that didn't seem to make any difference. Then I happened to come across a self-help book about eating disorders, and learned about bulimia – that people controlled their weight by throwing up their food. I started throwing up after meals and discovered I could eat what I wanted and lose weight. When I went to university at 18, I started starving myself through the day, making sure I was eating no more than 800 calories, then gorging myself in the evenings and throwing up. I knew I was out of control by this time, but I was slim, so it seemed worth it.

By the time I had left university, I had also started abusing laxatives very badly – taking 40 to 50 a day. I had to stay in every night as, not to put too fine a point on it, I couldn't be far away from a toilet. It also meant I couldn't have a full-time job.

In the end, I made a decision to stop doing this as I was simply bored of my life revolving around food and getting rid of it. But, of course, as it was the first time my body had been given food properly in years, it held onto it, and my weight ballooned, which I found very frightening.

I kept complaining to my boyfriend at the time about how much I hated being fat, and he would say, 'Do something about it then – join a gym'. Then I was made redundant from my job, so I did just that – I used the money to join a gym, and I absolutely fell in love with exercise.

I loved Tae Kwon do right from the start – it became a passion almost immediately. I liked the fact that it was a skill, and an on-going challenge. It seemed very different from simply working out in a gym.

It made me feel great. I realized at last that I had found the answer to weight control. If I exercised I could eat what I wanted without putting on weight. It was a revelation. I was still fairly big, but I didn't care anymore because I was fit and toned and happy for the first time in years. The final breakthrough came when I met Tessa and discovered my love of martial arts.

I took more fitness qualifications and eventually started personal training and working part-time at the Academy, a martial arts-based gym. It opened my eyes to a whole range of martial arts and I loved working there. At the same time, however, I felt there was a gulf between the people who came to the gym to do hard-core martial arts and those who came to do aerobics. There was no in-between, and this was when the idea for developing a hybrid of the two started to form.

When I left to do full-time personal training, I decided to introduce some martial arts moves as a way of offering clients new challenges and keeping the training fresh. They all loved it – they loved the fantasy of doing the kind of moves that you see in stunt scenes in the movies, and women in particular liked to punch and be given the permission to be angry. And, as there was no combat involved – the punches and kicks are aimed at a focus pad – it did not have the intimidating element which sometimes stops women doing a pure martial art. I kept the focus on perfecting the moves, rather than being aggressive. I also started to introduce moves from Tai Chi and Chi Gong, softer forms of martial arts, which are good for posture and relaxation.

I also discovered that training my clients this way got results much faster than normal training, which I put down to the mental focus involved –

as you have to concentrate on the moves, you don't notice how hard you're working, so you keep going longer. Kick boxing is particularly good for lengthening and toning muscles as the moves are about speed and endurance – it allows you to create a very athletic-looking figure.

> I knew I was onto something amazing when one of my clients went down from a size 16 to size 10 in less than 12 months.

She had never thought of herself as sporty before and now she was kicking and punching like a champion. Another 45-year-old businessman lost his beer gut then went on to do his black belt in kick boxing. It also had an amazing effect on an 11-year-old with learning difficulties – it improved her hand-eye coordination, balance and focus immensely.

WHY NOW?

I am not claiming that this style of training is unique. Unless you've been living on the moon, you'll have noticed that martial arts-based exercise routines have become the trendiest way to work out. In fact, martial arts and derivatives of martial arts have swept the USA and UK over the past two years, with exercisers of all ages and abilities falling in love with this style of fitness.

> For many people it is the first time in their lives they have been able to stick at one form of exercise, because they actually look forward to doing it. Exercisers all over the world who have embraced this technique are discovering that the benefits go far beyond firmer thighs and a flatter stomach – they feel stronger, less stressed and more confident in all areas of their lives.

But why have these ancient forms of exercise become so popular in the West now? To answer this we need to look at a little history. It's hard to believe that until 50 years ago formal exercise was virtually unheard of in this country outside of the army. It wasn't until after the Second World War that the BBC started broadcasting early morning keep-fit classes on the radio and urging the nation to 'stop slumping' in an effort to muster national morale. Keep-fit classes started springing up in local church halls, although it took another 20 years before the first gyms with specially-made equipment started to appear. But exercise remained a minority activity until the '80s, when Jane Fonda appeared on the scene and released her now infamous exercise video, urging us to 'go for the burn' while wearing Lycra and legwarmers. The aerobics boom began, closely followed by the birth of Step and, for the first time, women (and men other than boxers or body builders) were flocking to gyms.

It wasn't until the mid to late '90s that the exercise industry took time to stop and reflect on what all this activity was achieving. A whole gym-going generation had grown up and people were no longer happy to exercise for exercise's sake alone. So, in tune with the whole post-'80s approach to finding meaning in life, exercisers were looking for activities that not only got them in shape, but also enhanced their lives in other ways. Instead of 'going for the burn', we began looking for balance and total wellbeing in body and mind.

As it slowly dawned on us in the West that mind and body are intricately connected, we turned to the East, where this concept has been a central belief to many cultures for centuries. We 'discovered' the power of yoga to condition the body and mind from the inside out. The next logical step was to embrace the Eastern techniques known as martial arts, for their emphasis on mindfulness and being present in the 'here and now', on achieving balance and spiritual growth, as well as keeping the physical body in peak condition.

Until recently, the fitness industry in the Western world has recognized the mental benefits of exercise, but not really probed into it too

In martial arts, exercisers of the new millennium have found a way of keeping fit that also offers them a skill to learn and a progressive challenge that they can work towards – in short, exercise with meaning.

deeply. Any psychological benefits have tended to be explained by 'the exercise high' – the rush of endorphins (the brain's feelgood chemicals) into the bloodstream. But for centuries, Eastern cultures have believed that physical activity has a more important role to play – it can improve confidence, concentration and self-image – and in the case of martial arts, can bring philosophy and spirituality into everyday life.

SELF-DEFENCE OR SELF-DEVELOPMENT?

At this point you may well be thinking, 'Spirituality? Philosophy? I thought martial arts were all about turning the body into a lethal weapon!'

Traditional martial arts training is centred on hand-to-hand combat, but it goes hand-in-hand with healing and spiritual development.

These two elements may seem conflicting to us in the Western world, but it makes more sense when we consider that many martial arts were developed by monks as a way of protecting wealthy monasteries from marauding hordes! Shaolin Kung-fu, for example, was developed by Buddhist monks of the famous Shaolin temple in Northern China, whose monks practised louhan boxing, an ancient martial form, to keep fit for their hours of meditation and to be able to protect their monastery.

Courtesy is one of the first and most obvious things that you notice when you start a martial art. It is evident from the moment you walk into the 'Dojo' or training area. Whatever the martial art, there is usually some form of bow or mark of respect as you walk into the room. It is done in order to mark the fact that you are moving into a different type of space, a space where the martial

art and its principles are paramount. Junior grades respect senior grades and obey their instruction immediately and without question, but senior grades also have the responsibility to instruct junior grades; to set as good an example in style, technique and attitude as possible.

Students bow to the instructor at the beginning of the session, and to the instructor and senior grades at the end. Students also bow to each other during various other parts of the lesson. What can feel unnatural at first soon becomes second nature. I have been known to bow to a senior student while doing a weekly supermarket trip! It was a natural mark of respect and happened before I realized it.

Integrity follows on naturally from courtesy. Gradually the challenges met within the martial art class start to reflect the little challenges that life loves to throw at you. Integrity must therefore mean carrying on (or trying to!) the whole-hearted commitment to accuracy, effort and respect in all parts of your life. It is not easy but it must at least be attempted.

Self-control is clearly an important requirement when you are throwing kicks and punches around with others in close vicinity. Self-control is about understanding that you hold another person's wellbeing and body in your trust. It is about using your skills wisely and not showing off in order to impress others!

Indomitable spirit means an inner decision not to be defeated by any difficulty. It will mean different things at different times in your life. But it is a very important aspect not just to martial arts, but to coping with everyday living.

Today, all martial arts teaching centres on five tenets: courtesy, integrity, perseverance, self-control and indomitable spirit.

While the style of exercising described in this book is not a pure martial art, there is still scope to apply these tenets for personal development of mind, body and spirit. Take the bow, for example: As well as a mark of respect, the bow serves the purpose of bringing the mind in focus at the beginning of a class; to collect one's thoughts and to recognize and acknowledge your strength and vulnerability; and to focus on doing your best throughout the session. If you feel silly bowing before a session, then a couple of minutes quiet contemplation can serve the same purpose. And working with integrity means working to 100 per cent of your ability every time you work out. This is the fastest way to see results and make the most of your exercise time. Only you know when you are giving your full attention and effort; so you will have to be your own master in your exercise sessions! And whatever the challenge, you will not succeed without perseverance and indomitable spirit.

THE BOTTOM LINE

OK, lesson over, let's get down to business. Let's face it, the main reason most of us buy a book like this one – or buy an exercise video or join a gym for that matter – is to lose weight, tone up and get in shape. Rest assured, if you follow the advice in the following chapters, this will happen! If you want to lose fat, improve your muscle tone, drop a dress size, or balance out a pear shape, you have made the right choice – this form of exercising can do all this and more.

Many of you reading this will be new to the world of exercise (welcome!). But many will also be veterans of other exercise styles. If you've done Step or cardio-funk, if you've power-walked, jogged, or clocked up hours on an exercise bike, and you're still no nearer to reaching your ideal body, you're no doubt feeling far from convinced at this point. If so, great – it's good to question and think for yourself – in fact, these are essential requirements for a good kick boxer! So don't just take my word for it, read the hard facts.

FOUR REASONS KICK-IT! WILL GET YOU IN YOUR BEST SHAPE EVER

1 Every workout is a total body experience!

Have you ever thought that if you could just get rid of your excess fat (particularly on your bottom/thighs/stomach) you'd have the perfect body? Sound familiar? Then you think, if I go running/do aerobics/use my exercise bike every day I will burn off all the fat. And it doesn't work, does it? You give up long before you achieve your goal.

Apart from being boring, that approach to weight-loss is unbalanced. Achieving your best ever body is about more than just burning fat – you also need to strengthen your muscles and increase your flexibility. If you concentrate solely on burning fat, you'll end up with a smaller version of your existing body. You'll have the same imbalances, and they may even be exaggerated (pear-shaped women find this in particular – they tend to lose more weight from their upper body so the pear-shape becomes more pronounced). Balance is the key to achieving your best-ever body – combining fat-burning (cardiovascular work, which also conditions your heart and lungs) with strength and flexibility work. This will lengthen muscles that are too short, strengthen those that are weak and improve your posture.

Muscle imbalances are often the reason why women find it so hard to get that elusive flat stomach.

They think it's simply a case of having too much tummy fat (and of course, this can be a reason), but often they have a muscle imbalance problem, such as weak lower back muscles, allowing the tummy to stick out and look bigger than it is.

If you're thinking it's hard enough fitting cardiovascular work into a busy schedule, never mind strength and flexibility, you're not wrong! Which is why this work-out is so effective – it does all three at once.

The mix of kicks and punches looks deceptively easy, but is excellent at raising your heart-rate which is essential for burning calories – keep it up at a fast pace for more than a minute, and I guarantee you'll start to sweat.

At the same time, it provides resistance for your muscles which will help build lean muscle tissue, and this will help you lose weight too (the more lean muscle tissue you have, the higher your metabolic rate). You don't have to lift weights to build muscle tone – this routine uses your own bodyweight as resistance. Plus, because you're putting your muscles through a full range of movement (how many other exercise routines include hip-height side and front kicks?), you will improve your flexibility, which will encourage a long, lean look. All this in three 45-minute sessions a week!

It targets both the upper and lower body

When it comes to body image, men and women are at opposite ends of the spectrum. Most women are obsessed with their bottom halves, while men are fixated with their upper bodies. But in both cases, focussing on one body part to the exclusion of the rest is a recipe for disappointment. In men, the classic scenario is the over built-up chest on top of a weedy pair of legs; in women, it's an over-muscled lower half (thanks to endless Step and aerobics classes), with a neglected, untoned torso. The Kick-It! routines detailed in the following chapters are designed to target upper and lower body equally.

After all, your body is a sum of all its parts. If you're a pear-shaped woman, the most effective way of rebalancing your body is to take the focus off those dreaded hips and thighs, and think about adding some upper body definition – this will reduce the 'pear-shape' effect *and* boost your metabolic rate which will help to burn fat from your lower half. If you're worried about that developing beer gut, endless sit-ups aren't the answer. You need to get your whole body moving to burn off your excess fat, and that six-pack requires strong back muscles as much as strong stomach muscles.

Incidentally, women who can't read the word 'muscle' without worrying that they will end up looking like an East European shot-putter need not panic! You will not bulk up – it is actually very hard to increase muscle size, as all those men who have been trying to build up their chest for years will testify. Body builders achieve bulging muscles by lifting very heavy weights on a regular basis (amongst other things). This workout, by contrast,

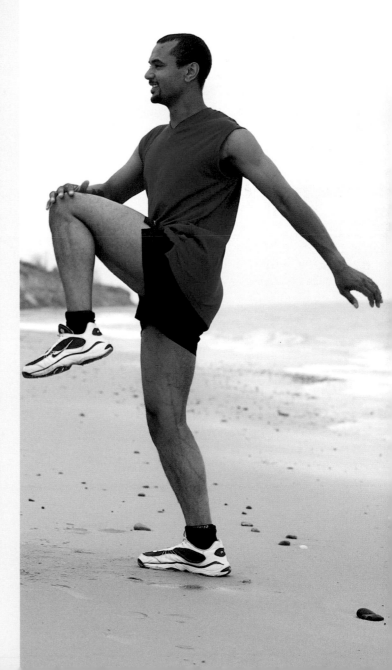

will encourage the development of long, lean, elegantly sculpted muscles (and trust me, men – *this* is what women find attractive. They are *not* turned on by a man with such overdeveloped pecs he looks like he should wear a bra!).

3   It's a mix of high and low impact

You don't need to be a rocket scientist to work out the difference between high and low impact exercise. High impact exercise involves the body leaving the ground so that when it makes contact a considerable force is jolted through the bones, joints and muscles. In low impact exercise the body does not leave the ground, so this force is eliminated.

Although high impact exercise (such as aerobics and jogging) has received bad press in terms of causing injuries, particularly of the knees and shins, it does have a role to play and it is important to have both types of impact in your exercise routine. High impact exercise is the most effective way to raise your heart-rate and therefore burn calories, but it is also vital for building strong bones. The jolt or shock that runs through your bones when you make impact with the ground when jumping or running causes your body to increase bone density. This is particularly important for women who can be at risk of osteoporosis, brittle-bone disease, in later life. But because excessive high impact exercise can lead to knee, lower back and shin pain, the ideal exercise routine, like Kick-It!, mixes high and low impact moves rather than relying on high impact alone. So this means that it works, but it doesn't hurt!

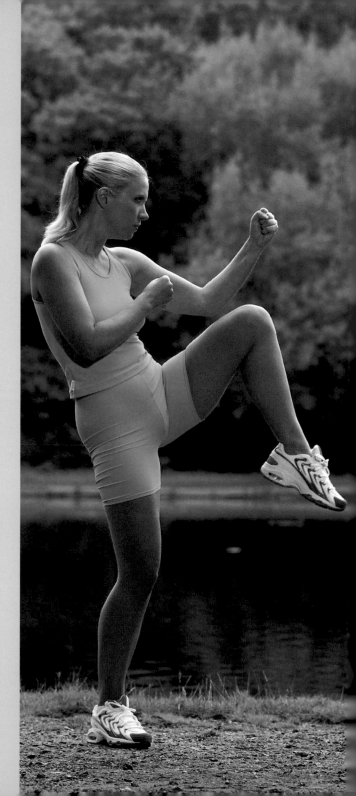

4 It's an interval workout

There's a commonly-held misconception that by working out at a moderate rate, we enter a magic 'fatburning zone' where we use mainly fat, rather than sugar, as fuel. While it is true that the body uses a higher *percentage* of fat for fuel at a moderate rate of activity, it is also true that it uses the highest percentage of fat for fuel when we're lying immobile, and everyone knows that you don't lose weight by lying down! So the thing to remember is that when it comes to weight-loss, it's total calorie expenditure that counts. If you did 30 minutes of moderate exercise, you'd burn around 150 calories (depending on your bodyweight). Push yourself as hard as you can and you'll burn around 350 calories in half an hour. Although your body will have used principally sugar for fuel, you will have created a 350 calorie deficit that your body will have to make up for later – by burning off fat.

The problem is, of course, that few of us can sustain a high level of activity for extended periods – and nor should we, as this is the surest way to get injured. But what we can do is interperse short periods of high level activity with periods of 'active recovery', keeping our heart-rate up but allowing us to feel comfortable enough to exercise for a longer period. This is known as interval training and is used by all athletes to improve their fitness. The Kick-It! routines are also interval training as they mix heart-rate raising routines such as kicks and punches with less strenuous moves such as squats and lunges.

BUT…

Ready to get going? Or have you got a question or two you'd like answering first, a few 'Buts'? I thought so! While I can't read your mind in particular, I do have answers to the most common concerns and queries that people have when they're introduced to this style of exercising for the first time:

1 But I'm unco-ordinated!

The key is to spend enough time on chapter 3, *Mastering the Basics*, before you move on to the workouts themselves. Each move is broken down into detailed step-by-step instructions. You can't practise these too much. If you're standing at the bus-stop or in the queue for the supermarket checkout, go through the moves in your head (those of us who are of a particularly uninhibited disposition can do the moves themselves).

Let me tell you now that you will not be good at most of these moves from day one. (Unless you're a natural, in which case you should think about giving up the day job and taking up kick boxing professionally). These are skilful moves and you will improve with time and this is partly what makes the workout effective – you will not 'plateau' (reach a point where you stop seeing results) like you do with other exercise routines. The better you get at these moves, the more power you can put into your kicks and punches and therefore the more benefits you will see.

2 But I'm not aggressive!

It's a common misconception that martial arts are about aggression. I admit it's one that is easily made – a lot of kickboxers look like they eat small children for breakfast when they're competing. In fact, as mentioned earlier, the ancient Eastern traditions behind martial arts are about achieving spiritual growth and balance rather than beating the living daylights out of your opponent. So you don't need an aggressive nature to feel comfortable with this technique.

That said, Kick-It! is an effective way of relieving stress, and if you *want* to imagine that your boss's face is on the receiving end of one of your roundhouse kicks, there's nothing to stop you!

3 But I'm very unfit!

Then you've taken the first step to becoming fitter. This routine can be adapted to any level of fitness and is safe for all ages and levels of fitness. But be sure to fill in the health-screen questionnaire in chapter 2, *Getting Started* first.

4 But I need to lose so much weight, I don't know where to begin!

Begin by turning the page and changing your life. Don't think of this as a necessary evil that must be endured so you can fit into that dress or swimsuit. This is the beginning of a permanent lifestyle change. And trust me, you are going to look back and wonder why you waited so long! See chapter 10, *10 Tips for a Healthy Lifestyle*, for further guidance.

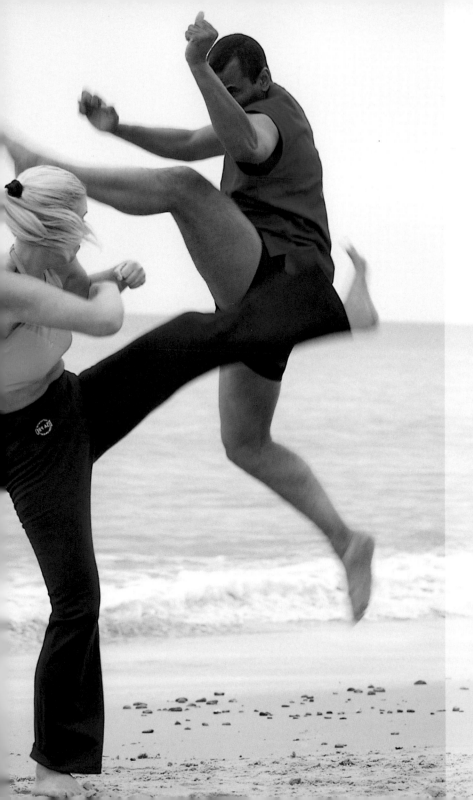

5 But I don't have time to exercise!

This is the most common excuse given for not exercising. And I'm sorry to sound unsympathetic, but I simply do not believe it. We make time for the things that we want in our lives and if you truly want to get fit, you will make time for it. It might involve getting up earlier, cutting down on your TV watching or giving up an evening in the pub, but if you want to do it, you'll find a way. See chapter 2 for more tips on how to make exercise a habit.

So, no more 'Buts' – it's time to kick butt!

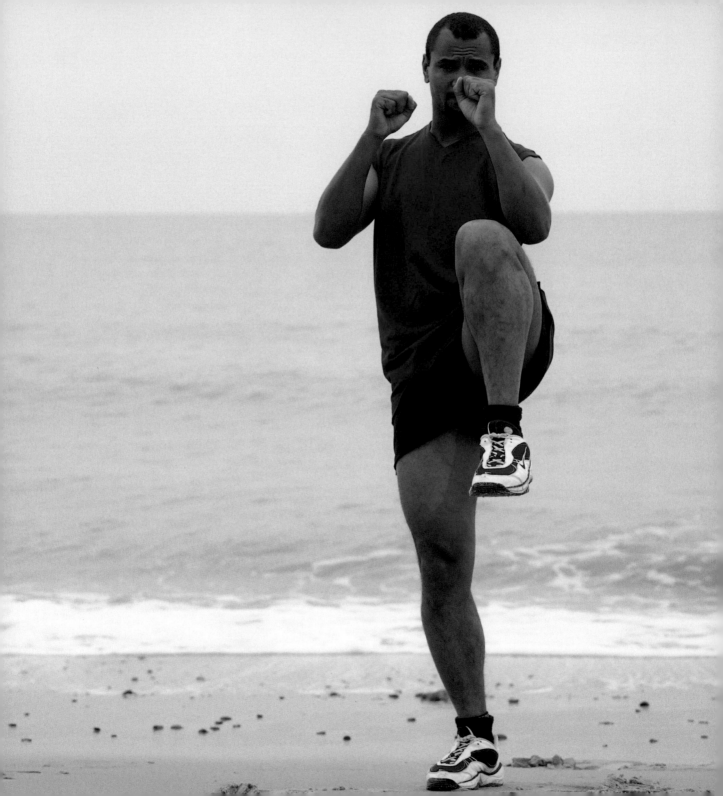

GETTING STARTED

Before you go any further, it's essential that you complete the following questionnaires to find out if you are fit to work out. For the majority of the population, exercise improves health and wellbeing, but a minority should only exercise under supervision from their doctor. It's also very important not to ignore any past or present injuries or niggling muscle or joint pains. Pain is always a message from the body that something is wrong, and it will invariably get worse, rather than better, with exercise. However, the source of such problems is often very simple and can be corrected – it doesn't mean you have to resign yourself to a life of pain or inactivity.

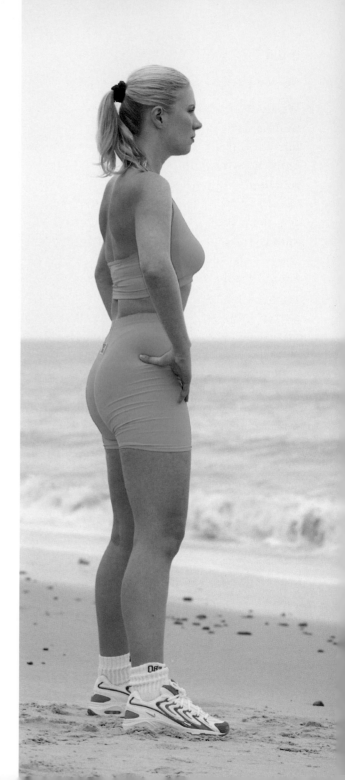

QUESTIONNAIRE 1

Do you need to see a doctor?

Consult your medical practitioner before starting this or any other exercise routine if you answer 'Yes' to any of the questions below. (If you don't answer yes to any of the questions below, but still have doubts about your health, it is wise to consult a doctor anyway).

1 Have you ever been diagnosed with a heart condition, or is there a history of heart disease in the family?

2 Are you more than three stone (42lbs) overweight?

3 Do you have high blood pressure?

4 Are you diabetic?

5 Are you asthmatic or do you have a history of breathing problems?

6 Are you pregnant or trying to become pregnant?

7 Have you recently given birth?

8 Have you had surgery in the last six weeks?

9 Have you recently experienced chest pain during physical activity?

10 Have you ever been advised by a doctor to avoid exercise?

QUESTIONNAIRE 2

Do you need to see a physiotherapist?

We tend to view physiotherapists and related professionals such as osteopaths and chiropractors as people to turn to when we're injured or in pain. However, they have an equally important role to play in preventing us becoming injured in the first place. There is nothing more demotivating than starting an exercise routine full of enthusiasm and commitment only to be stalled a few weeks later by a recurring knee, back or shoulder pain. It's at this point that the exercising sceptics will chip in and say, 'See, I knew exercise was bad for you!' The point is that exercise is not bad for you, but modern life *is* bad for your body. Most of us force our bodies to do actions that they were not designed to do for hours at a time: sitting hunched over a computer or a steering wheel, for instance, or simply carrying a heavy bag on one shoulder. The end result is a body that we have become used to as normal, but which is invariably imbalanced. Overuse of some muscles while underuse of others creates imbalances that can result in joints being pulled out of alignment. Many people will eventually suffer pain from these imbalances during everyday life, but exercise will escalate the rate at which problems occur because it places increased force on joints and muscles.

A good physiotherapist will check out your body and let you know if you have any imbalances that could lead to problems, along with ways to eliminate them (usually rehabilitative exercises or sometimes, in the case of lower body problems, specially developed shoe inserts). Most gyms or your GP can recommend physios. You should definitely seek a consultation if you answer 'yes' to any of the questions below:

Do you ever suffer from knee pain (e.g. when walking downstairs)?

Have you ever had shin splints?

Do you suffer from lower back problems?

Do you suffer regular 'twinges' in your shoulders or upper back muscles?

Have you ever been told not to exercise for any length of time by a relevant professional e.g. physiotherapist?

Do you have bunions or other foot problems?

Have you ever fractured or broken any bones?

Have you ever had surgery on a joint or ligaments (e.g. after a skiing accident)?

WHAT TO WEAR

Clothes wise, wear what you feel comfortable in and what will allow you a full range of movement. Many of the big sportswear brands such as Nike, Adidas and USAPro are producing ranges with loose-fitting trousers and T-shirts that are ideal. Don't go for anything too baggy, however – or your movements will be hindered by too much fabric.

It is vital that you do these workouts while wearing the right trainers to protect your body from injury. Choose a cross trainer or a shoe designed for use in studio classes or for gym work rather than a running shoe. You need good cushioning in the forefront and the heel, to lessen the impact during jumping, plus a design that offers lateral stability (in other words, support for the sides of the feet to help you balance during kicks and other moves.) You don't have to spend a fortune – you should be able to get a pair for under £70 ($100). Unfortunately, many sports stores don't have trained assistants to advise you in buying trainers, and many of us simply make our choice on looks alone. If there isn't an assistant in the store who can help you, then opt for a gym or studio shoe or a cross trainer, go for a low rather than a high (ankle boot) cut, and make sure you try the trainer on and walk around the store in it (better still, jump up and down in it!) You may need the next size up from your usual shoe size to make sure you have plenty of toe room as feet swell during exercise.

WHERE TO EXERCISE

The beauty of Kick-It! is that you can do it anywhere. I have a client who does her exercise routine in her local park. She sometimes ends up with an audience of mesmerized children, but she is so extrovert, she doesn't care. She is the exception to the rule, however – I think it's safe to say that most of us prefer to exercise in the privacy of our own homes. Because this routine is mostly done on the spot, you don't need a huge amount of space, and you don't need any equipment. That means you can do it in your hotel room when you're travelling, in your garden in the summer – even in your bathroom if this is the only room in your house where you can lock the door against inquisitive children (or housemates). Many people find it helps to have some motivating music to work out to, and a full-length mirror is useful for checking technique. You will need a skipping rope for the fat-burning workout (around £10 ($15) from sports stores and department stores – opt for a lightweight plastic rope) and a mat or towel for the abdominal work. Apart from that, all you need is a glass of water to sip throughout the workout.

WHEN TO EXERCISE

Just what is the best time of day to work out? It's a subject of debate among sports scientists. It is commonly thought that strength and endurance peak in the late afternoon, coinciding with the highest body temperature. The majority of sport records are broken at this time of day. The only problem is, of course, that most of us are at work in the late afternoon.

What about first thing in the morning? Some sports scientists believe that exercising at this time in the morning revs up the metabolic rate so that you burn calories all day, and others believe that exercising in the morning before breakfast (i.e. on an empty stomach) forces the body to use fat for fuel. But if you're not a morning person, however motivated you feel to get in shape, you'll ignore the alarm when it goes off at 6.30am and consequently feel like a failure all day. You may even give up exercise altogether thinking, 'I just can't stick to it.' But in this case, you're being too hard on yourself – lots of committed exercisers say they could never do an early morning workout! But there are others, however, for whom this time of day is perfect – their energy levels are at their highest and they can guarantee time to themselves without work or social commitments intervening.

After a day at work – even if you're desk-bound – you can feel so tired that it's a huge effort to simply drag yourself home and collapse on the sofa. The last thing you need is to do some exercise, right? Wrong! Believe it or not, a workout will energize you, as it is an outlet for the tension you have accumulated in mind and body throughout the day. Exercising after work can leave you feeling relaxed and refreshed and in a much better position to enjoy your evening – it's a much more effective de-stresser than knocking back several glasses of wine. So, the trick is to experiment and find the best time for you. You may even surprise yourself by discovering the pre-breakfast you!

Having pinpointed your optimal exercise time, you then need to work out if it is feasible to exercise at this time. It may well be that it isn't – you may feel at your best at lunchtime, for instance, but have a job where a lunchtime workout is out of the question. But if your job is a little more flexible, then consider joining a nearby gym and doing your Kick-It! workouts in a quiet corner (and take it from me, no-one will think you're strange and stare at you – people in gyms are too busy looking at themselves in the mirror to worry about what anyone else is up to). Many committed lunch-hour exercisers say that it not only makes the working day go faster, it eliminates the mid-afternoon slump.

It really is a case of finding the right time of day to exercise. Ideally, you should choose the time when you feel at your best, because this is when you'll do the best workout.

LET'S GET MOTIVATED!

Recognize the following scenario? 'I start a new exercise routine full of enthusiasm. I've lost count of the number of times I've joined a gym, or spent money on equipment. But it's always the same – after about six weeks, I start to lose interest, and before I know it, I've stopped exercising altogether. Maybe I should just give up trying to get fit.' If it sounds familiar, you're not alone – an estimated 75 per cent of new gym members stop going regularly after six weeks.

There are endless convincing reasons to keep fit – it gets you in shape, reduces stress and helps you feel more confident. OK, so if you know all the benefits, why it is so hard to make it a regular part of your life? Well, for lots of reasons: it's time-consuming, hard, takes a long time to make a difference, etc. But it's also more complex than that.

Psychologists have identified five different stages that lead to exercise becoming a regular part of your life. In the first stage, called pre-contemplation, a person is unaware of and uninterested in exercise. Stage two is contemplation, when the person is aware of the benefits of exercise but hasn't taken any action yet. The next stage, preparation, is when the decision to exercise has been made and the person has made contact with a gym or club (or bought a book like this one). Then comes activity, learning the ropes, setting and achieving goals and keeping to a routine. After that we reach the maintenance stage, when exercise becomes part of your life. Tackling these stages gradually means the hurdles to exercising will fade as the benefits take over. But expecting to suddenly go from doing nothing at all to being a five-times-a-week exerciser is a tall order, and one that most of us fail to meet – hence the six week drop-out.

But you should also be aware that relapse and drop-out are a fact of exercise life and acknowledging this ebb and flow is vital. You can't maintain the same intensity of commitment permanently. There will be times when you want to make exercise more of a priority in your life than others. Accepting this and not feeling guilty or a failure because of it is vital, as is changing your perception of what qualifies as exercise. Sometimes you will be happy to fit structured sessions into your life three to five times a week. Other times, simply being more active throughout your day is enough. Accept this natural ebb and flow and you will begin to let go of the feelings of guilt and failure that you associate with exercise.

EXERCISE FOR THE RIGHT REASONS

Exercising for the right reasons is the key to sticking at it long term. According to psychologists, there are two types of motivation. Extrinsic motivation is driven by outside factors – exercising because you hate the way your bottom looks in the mirror, or because your friends do it, or because your partner has been making jibes about you putting on weight. While these motives can work well at first, they will stop doing so after a while because you are exercising under sufferance.

What exercisers who stick at it long term have in common is intrinsic motivation – exercising because you want to, because you know and physically feel how it improves your wellbeing and quality of life. That means you've stopped comparing yourself with other people and dreaming that when you've exercised enough to get the perfect body, all your problems will melt away; you've realized that while exercising might not give you a perfect body, it can give you the best version of your own body; that it can also give you increased energy, a sense of centre and balance, a new perspective on life and a feeling of strength. Exercisers with intrinsic motivation see exercise as one of life's joys rather than a chore.

But don't despair if you feel miles away from reaching this state of mind. Studies have shown that most exercisers start off with extrinsic motivation, and gradually develop intrinsic motivation. And, in the initial stages, be aware that lots of other factors will influence your likelihood of moving on, which we will look at in greater detail later in this chapter.

SET REASONABLE GOALS

It's easy to be discouraged when your expectations are wildly unrealistic. After all, if your goal is to lose weight to look like Kate Moss or Pierce Brosnan, it'll be no surprise when you give up after six weeks because you don't see that – even if you do see a slimmer, fitter version of yourself. Effective goals are realistic, measurable and specific and flexible, and there is even research to prove this. Psychologist Dr Fiona James of the University of Hertfordshire, studied 115 people on a 12 week exercise programme. All were asked to rate how they imagined they'd feel at the end of the programme in terms of body size, confidence, health and happiness and stress levels. Those who finished the course tended to expect small changes relating to weight loss and health, but those who dropped out had higher expectations concerning wider areas of their life, such as happiness and confidence. The researchers concluded that you must not expect an exercise programme to change your life.

Women in particular set themselves very high standards to live up to. A man with an average body will look at himself in the mirror and think, 'I'm not half bad, you know'. A woman with an average body will look at herself in the mirror and think, 'Ugh, those thighs. The size of my bottom.' Women tend to home in on faults and ignore good points, or fail to see faults as part of the overall big picture of the body. Women also tend to blame themselves for these perceived faults – they stare at their thighs and think that if they didn't have such a weakness for pizza, chocolate cake or Australian Chardonnay, they'd have the thighs of a ballet dancer (while conveniently ignoring the fact that their mother and sisters have the same thighs as they do). Yes, it's a sad fact of life that the way our body looks is largely down to genetics. But, before you throw this book away and think, 'Well what's the point of exercising, then?', you *can* improve it and have *your* best ever body. It's amazing how liberating it is to know that you are doing the best by your body and your health. You can look at the naturally skinny-minnie or muscle-bound hunk on the beach and think, 'Well, I'll never look like that but I know that I look my best', and that can be very satisfying (and bear in mind that that skinny-minnie or hunk probably goes home and agonizes at some perceived faults in the mirror as well!).

Getting in shape and improving your health inside and out will benefit your life in a multitude of ways, but it isn't a magic bullet and it won't dissolve all your problems. If you hate your job, you will hate it whether you are size 14 or a size 10. If you want a boyfriend or girlfriend, you still have to get out and meet people whether or not you have the perfect body! But what improving the way you feel about your body *can* do is give you the confidence to change your life and achieve your dreams.

WRITE A MISSION STATEMENT

Once you've decided on your goal, write it down as your own personal mission statement. OK, it may sound like New Age psycho-babble, but if multimillion dollar businesses around the world think it works, there must be something in it. After all, it's simply common sense that you can't achieve a goal without knowing what that goal is in the first place! Your personal mission statement should set out in black and white, why you have decided to exercise; what it will bring to your life that you don't already have; and how it will change the way you look and feel. It may take you a few gos to get it right and don't worry about feeling silly; no-one but you needs to read it, so be frank and honest with yourself.

Once you're happy with your mission statement, write it out and keep it where you can read it whenever you feel your motivation waning. Here are a few examples:

- 'I want to tone up my legs so that I can stop hiding them in trousers when I really want to wear skirts like my friends. I want to walk into a clothes shop and buy what I like the look of, not what will cover up my body.'
- 'I want to feel strong and fit and in control in my life. I want to

know that I could kick someone hard if they attacked me. I want to stop feeling guilty about not exercising.'

- 'I want to make exercise part of my life because I want to stop feeling scared of getting old.'

- 'I want to work at reducing my stress levels because I know that at the moment they are too high. I want to find a way of relaxing that I enjoy.'

- 'I want to lose my unhealthy habits like eating the wrong things, smoking and drinking too much. I want to get fit to make this easier.'

- 'I want to lose weight so that the next time I see my ex, he realizes just what he's missing!'

You may want to update your mission statement at regular intervals as your fitness level and your goals change. For example, statements like the last one may no longer seem important and you'll be exercising for you, not to make a point to others.

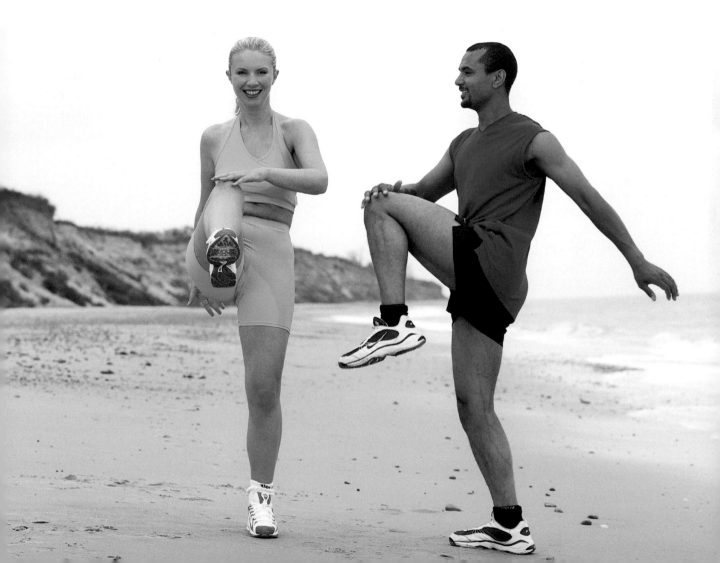

KEEP A TRAINING DIARY

Next to a good pair of trainers, a training diary is your most important piece of fitness equipment. Like a food diary, which is a very revealing way to learn what you actually eat as opposed to what you think you eat, a training diary will show you how often you exercise, and will motivate you to exercise more. You can buy special training diaries from sports shops (they are particularly popular with runners), but an ordinary diary will do just as well. On the days you don't exercise, put a cross. On the days that you do exercise, put a tick. Before long, you'll be making sure there are more ticks than crosses. Then record how long you exercised for, what you did and how you felt (record any niggles such as knee or shoulder pain – if they recur it is worth seeing a physiotherapist to get them checked out). Record if you found an exercise hard. It can be very motivating to look back and see how easy you find an exercise that you used to dread! It can be revealing to record next to your crosses why you chose not to exercise that day – a pattern may emerge that can indicate a need to address an aspect of your lifestyle – for instance, if you routinely miss workouts because of feeling hungover, you may want to look at your alcohol consumption.

Here's an example of a training diary entry:

MONDAY

Time: 45 minutes:

Workout: Lower body workout.

Notes: Got up early and did 45 minute workout before work. Felt great as had done nothing since Thursday and was really ready to work out. Felt like I really got the hang of the timing of those punches and kicks together. Felt relaxed and energized all day.

TUESDAY

X

Rest day

WEDNESDAY

X

Had planned to work out this evening but went to the pub after work instead. It was a boring evening and I spent too much money and ended up with a hangover. Next time I'll say no and do my workout instead.

THURSDAY

X

No workout due to hangover from Wednesday night. Felt tired all day.

FRIDAY

Time: 1 hour 30 minutes

Workout: Upper and lower body workout.

Was determined to make up for the rest of the week. Did extra long workout after work, with lots of cardio to burn off those alcohol calories and a good abs workout. Went to bed feeling very relaxed and slept like a baby.

IT'S ALL IN THE PLANNING!

Spontaneity is a wonderful thing, so why not just do your workouts when the urge takes you? There's nothing wrong with this – unless you want to see results of course! If you do want to get fitter and shape up, then you need to plan – on two levels. First, sit down at the start of every week and plan when are the best times to exercise. Then schedule them into your week by putting them in your diary, Psion organizer or kitchen wall calendar as you would any other appointment. Then stick to them.

The second level of planning involves each individual workout. For maximum effectiveness, simply deciding you're going to exercise isn't enough. You must decide how much time your session is going to last, how it will start, progress, and then end. In other words, choose which one or combination of workouts described in this book you are going to do. You may even want to write this down in your workout diary (see above), with boxes to tick off what you've done. It may seem time-consuming, but what you get is the benefits of having a personal trainer without having to pay for one. It means you're less likely to give up halfway through a workout – when you know you have a set number of moves to do, even if you're not in the mood to work out, you can see the end of the tunnel. It also is a way of working progressively and of making sure that you work all the muscle groups of the body.

BELIEVE IN YOURSELF

You're making a big and long-term lifestyle change by committing to exercising regularly. Don't underestimate that. You'll need all the help you can get, from friends, family and yourself. There's a lot of truth in the saying that 'you can be your own worst enemy'. How many times have you looked at yourself in the mirror and said something along the lines of, 'You'll never be slim and fit. You're useless, you can't do anything'? Then, surprise, surprise, it isn't long before you abandon your good intentions once again. Think about those words: you would never be so cruel, negative and demotivating to a friend would you? So why do you allow that voice in your head to sabotage yourself so often?

Changing the very way you think can seem like the hardest task of all. But it isn't – it's just a question of habit. We like to think that as humans we are complex and fascinating beings but, in fact, we are a lot simpler than we realize. A lot of what we do simply comes down to habit, and habits are a lot easier to modify than we think. Next time that negative voice pops into your head, tell it to go away. Think of a positive alternative. Say, for instance, you're doing a roundhouse kick, you catch sight of yourself in the mirror and that voice says, 'Look at the size of those thighs. They're huge and they'll never be any thinner. I might as well give up now,' at this point you respond (in your head – or out loud if you prefer!), 'No! I am not as fit as I'd like to be but I am doing something about it. If I continue I will see results. I won't see improvements by giving up.'

Get into the habit of giving yourself positive self-talk and you will be amazed to discover before long that it *is* just a habit and not necessarily a symptom of deep psychological problems such as poor self-esteem. Anyone who's spent time with a weight-conscious friend can testify to the truth of this – you start with a robust, normal body image, but by the end of the holiday/working period with the person who is obsessed with calories and body fat, you find that you're beginning to obsess yourself. Once you've moved on and left that person behind, you realize that it was simply a phase, like taking on someone's style of dressing or taste in music.

Which is why it is of vital importance that you surround yourself with the right people. 'Toxic' friends will recognize that your efforts to start exercising are a good sign, but will try to undermine them. Perhaps they realize that once you are slim and fit you will have more confidence so will be less willing to be influenced by them. Maybe, as is often the case in a boyfriend or girlfriend, they are even scared that you will leave them. Parents can also be threatened by change in their children and be demotivating as a result. 'Oh, you'll never be slim,' your mother will say, 'not like your sister'. Most probably, she knows very well that you could be slim, but she's petrified that if you do lose weight, you'll have the confidence to travel round the world like your sister and then she won't have either of you nearby.

With toxic friends, you should weigh up what you get out of having them in your life. If you feel the benefits outweigh the negative comments, then tackle them by saying you are serious about getting fit and would appreciate their support. Why not enlist their help in some way – get them to phone you up on the days you have planned to work out to remind you – or better still, do your workouts with you. A similar approach could get family on board. It's amazing how people's attitude can change once they feel involved and needed. If this doesn't work, then the easiest way to cut out the negativity is to not tell them about your plans. Tell your hopes, plans and dreams to supportive people in your life only – and make sure that you yourself are one of those supportive people.

Don't give yourself a hard time. Failure is just an indication of where improvements can occur. If you have dropped out in the past, put it behind you, look to the future and ask, what do I want to achieve now? Don't waste energy hating yourself.

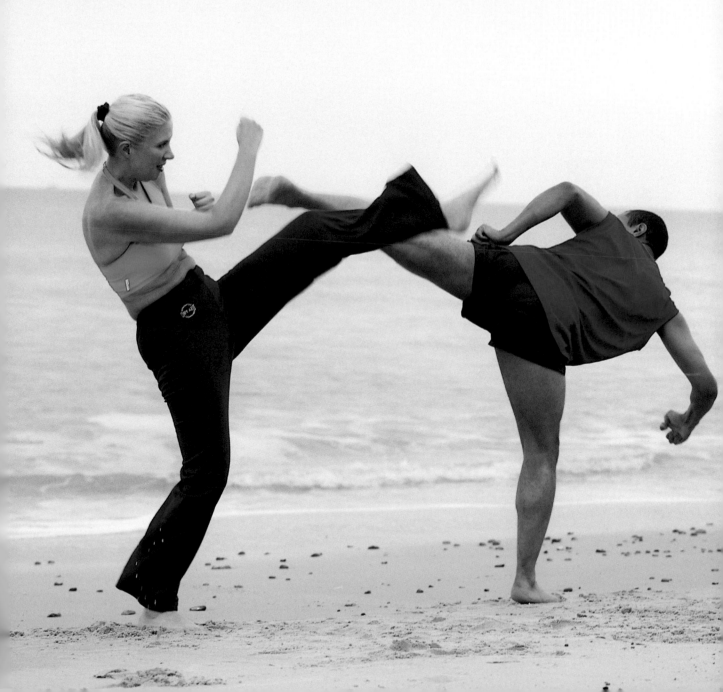

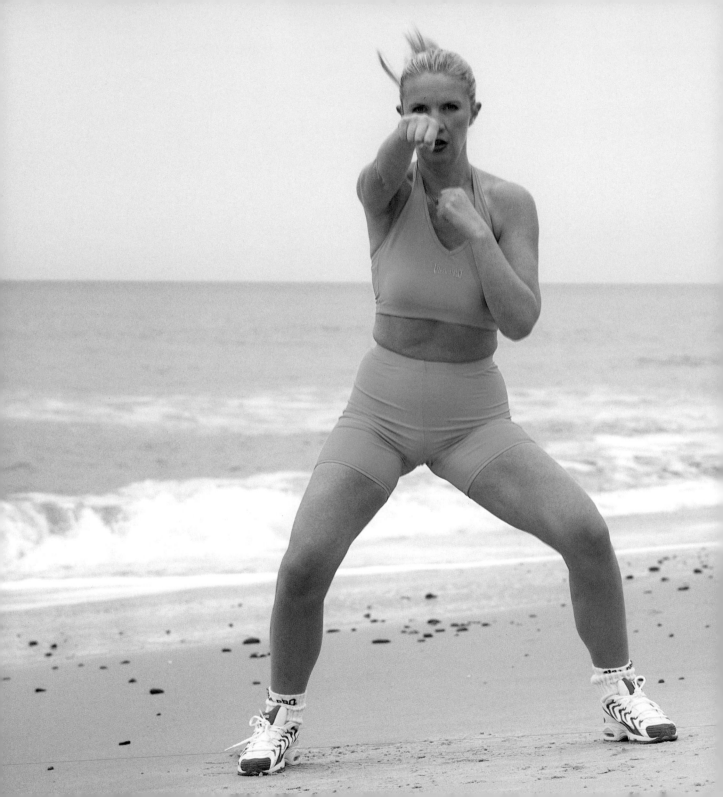

CHAPTER THREE

MASTERING THE BASICS

If you are anything like me, by now you'll be dying to get to the workouts themselves and are thinking you might just skip this chapter! Unfortunately, this is the worst thing you can do for many reasons. It may have been a long time since you kicked and punched – since you were a child perhaps? So you're not only having to engage your muscles in a way that will feel unfamiliar, but you are also having to engage your brain – more specifically, the neural pathways in your brain that tell your muscles what to do. Ever wondered why you can watch a move – whether in an exercise routine or while learning a new sport – believe that you have completely understood, only to be frustrated that you can't repeat it correctly yourself? That's because your brain is unused to sending the relevant signals to your muscles. Just like foot-paths on a country walk, the more the neural pathways are used, and the more established they become, the easier it is to do the moves you want to do correctly.

So it's vital that you spend enough time mastering the basics before you move onto the workouts to ensure your brain is fully on board and ready to take on the challenge of stringing the individual moves together in a sequence. Spending time on the basics will also improve the quality of your workout 100 per cent and, although you may be champing at the bit to get started, you will actually see results faster if you invest enough time at the beginning in getting the moves right.

Secondly, as any athlete knows, poor preparation leads to injury as well as disappointing performance. By recognizing that everything we do has natural stages – i.e. we learn to walk before we run – we are already mentally preparing ourselves to learn our basic skills properly. Picture an iceberg floating in the sea – the visible tip represents our workouts, the unseen remainder represents your preparation!

So exactly how long should you spend on this chapter? That will vary between individuals, but a good guide for most people is to spend 20 minutes a day on one or two of the basic moves a week, until you have covered all of them.

You will know when it is time to move on when you can work through the basic moves without needing the book for reference and you feel that you can flow through each move with ease. But it's always a good idea to put in some practice on individual moves at regular intervals to keep your technique precise.

TIPS TO MAKE IT WORK

Forget embarrassment

While practising, don't be put off by feeling that you look stupid! Failure is an integral part of everyone's learning process. In order to learn we have to be aware of what we are doing wrong. If you don't feel that you are getting it right, it really doesn't matter. Be aware of what you are getting wrong, don't tense up out of fear and embarrassment, and try again.

Use a friend

Working out with a buddy is a great motivator. Not only can you check each other's technique, but you also have a training partner who can inspire you on those days when you are looking for any old excuse not to exercise.

Use a mirror

You are not being vain staring at yourself in a mirror. Use the mirror as a tool to check your posture, stance, and technique. In fact always use a mirror whenever you have the chance – the bigger the better!

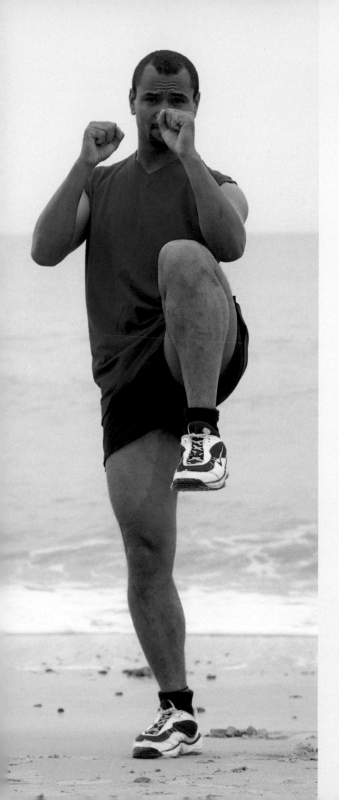

HOW TO MAKE A FIST

It sounds simple enough, but you'd be surprised at how different people's ideas of a fist can be! The fist used in martial arts training has the front part of the index and middle finger as its striking point.

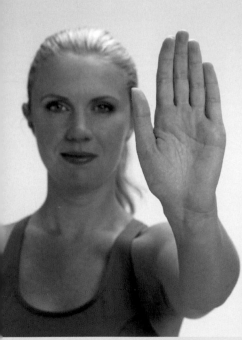

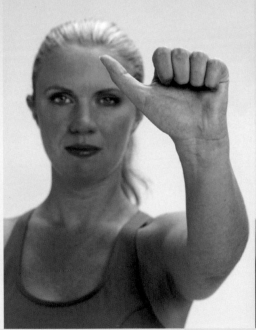

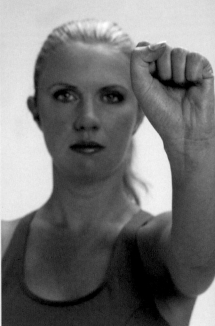

1 Hold your hand out with the palm flat.

2 Begin folding in from the tops of the fingers leaving out the thumb. Fold fingers over and clench them to the palm.

3 Place the thumb firmly on the four folded fingers.

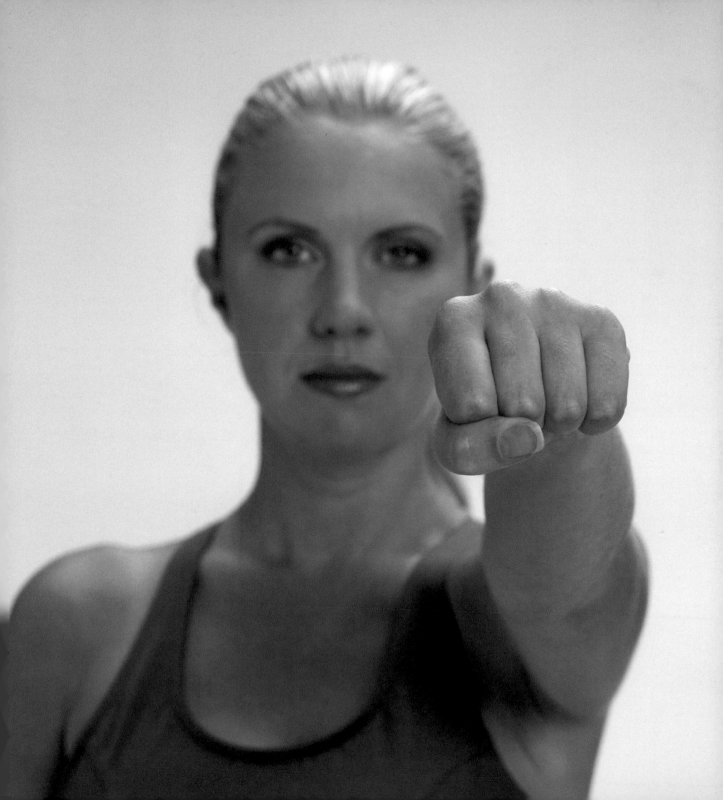

2 HOW TO STAND

The power of a punch comes from the body, not the hand, so before we learn to punch, we have to learn how to stand. Correct stances are the foundation stone for the rest of the techniques. They should make you feel in control, alert and ready to move.

Before you start, stand up and focus for a moment on your natural stance. Learning the stances is a bit like learning to stand up again, in that in many cases you will be doing the opposite of what comes naturally. Pay attention to your feet and knees – even when standing with straight legs your knees should be soft (i.e. not locked out). In martial arts, your weight should be forward on the ball of your foot, rather than through the heels.

It is important to master the stances because if contact with the floor is wrong, the position of the pelvis and angle of the spine will be wrong too, which will make it difficult to put power into any technique.

Your balance is also bound to be compromised if the distribution of weight between the feet is misplaced in any way. Keep your weight evenly distributed between each leg.

Finally, keep your abdominal muscles tight, with your ribcage lifted. Your neck should be straight and your shoulders back. Think of your abdominal region as your centre and keep it strong with a straight back and tight abs.

A Basic stance

For punches.

Stand with feet hip-width apart. Knees are soft and directly in line with your toes. Bottom is tucked under. Ribcage is lifted with the shoulders back and down. Hands are relaxed down the side of the body. Crown of the head is lifted with the chin slightly tucked in.

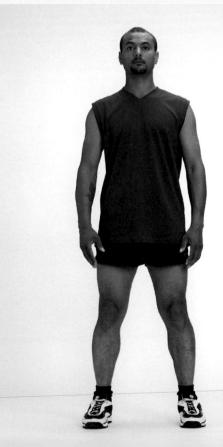

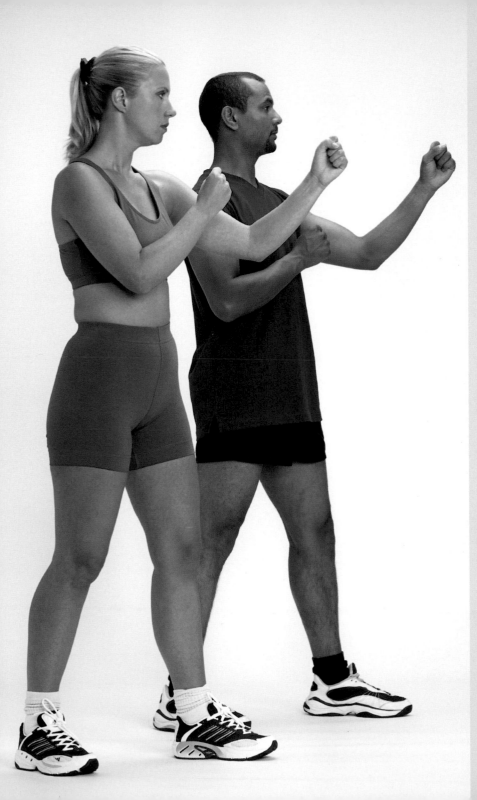

B Fighting stance

For punches and front kicks.

Stand sideways with your feet shoulder-width apart. Your front foot faces forward and your rear foot slightly outwards. Keep the weight distributed evenly on both legs. Make sure your knees are 'soft' and your weight on the ball of your foot. With closed fists and bent elbows, keep the arms close to the body. If the left leg is leading then the left bent arm should be in front with the elbow pointing downwards and the fist pointing up. The right arm lies across the chest with the elbow close to the body.

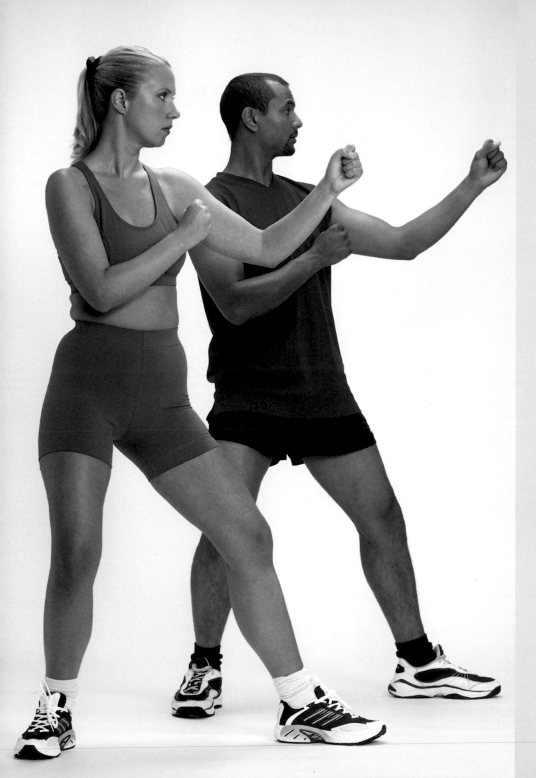

C Back stance

For turning kicks and side kicks.

This stance differs from the fighting stance in that the weight distribution is placed much more on the back leg, enabling you to lift up your front leg with ease. Legs are slightly further apart with the toes of the rear foot pointing outward or even slightly behind. Both knees are bent. Arms are the same as the fighting stance.

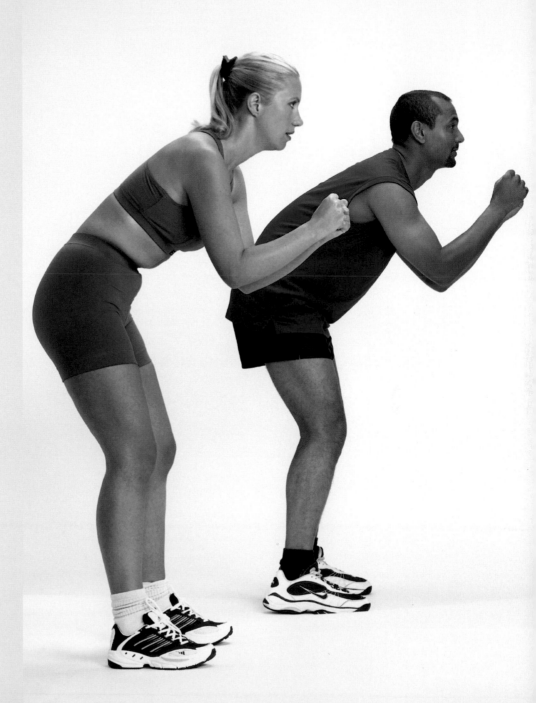

D Back kick stance

For back kicks.

With the feet no more than shoulder-width apart and the knees well bent, tilt the upper body forwards 25 degrees. Arms are up in front of chest. Make sure you keep your back straight.

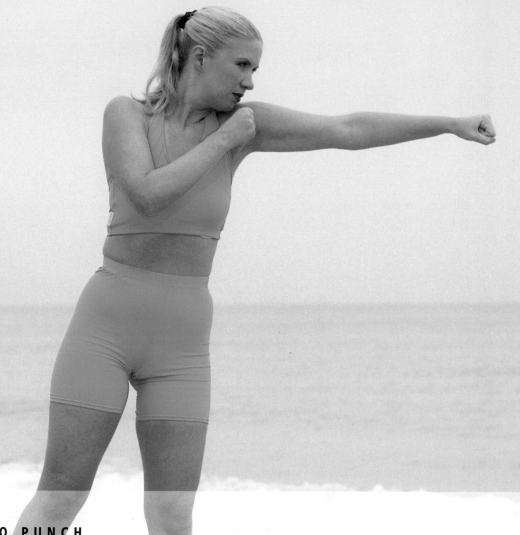

3 HOW TO PUNCH

Your fist should be strong and tight but not so tense that you feel any strain in your forearm or wrist. Never fully extend your arm so you are locking out any joints. Always give yourself a mental target when you punch. Think about punching a foot behind your target to make sure that you punch 'through' it.

Remember a punch is not just thrown from the arms and shoulders, it requires the correct whole body mechanics behind it to make it safe and effective. Make sure you keep your fist, wrist and elbow in perfect alignment i.e. an unbroken line throughout. Breathe out on every punch that you throw. Inhale as you retract.

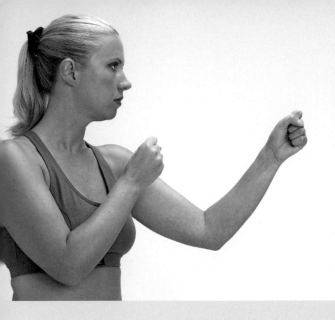
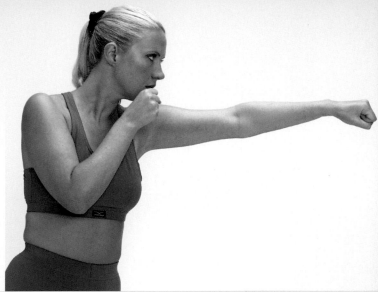

A Front hand punch or jab

From fighting stance.

The front arm punch is a small movement. The action begins in the hips and when the punch is released the bodyweight is brought forward onto the bent front leg. The punching shoulder swings freely behind the punch. Retract the punch quickly.

B Back hand punch or cross

From fighting stance.

The back hand punch begins with a hip twist which drives the punching hand forwards and the back heel off the floor. This brings the weight forward onto the bent front leg. Bring the arm back to the original position.

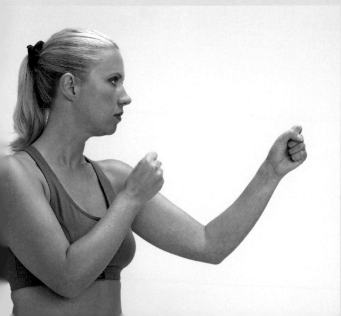
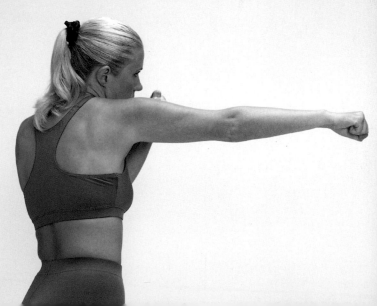

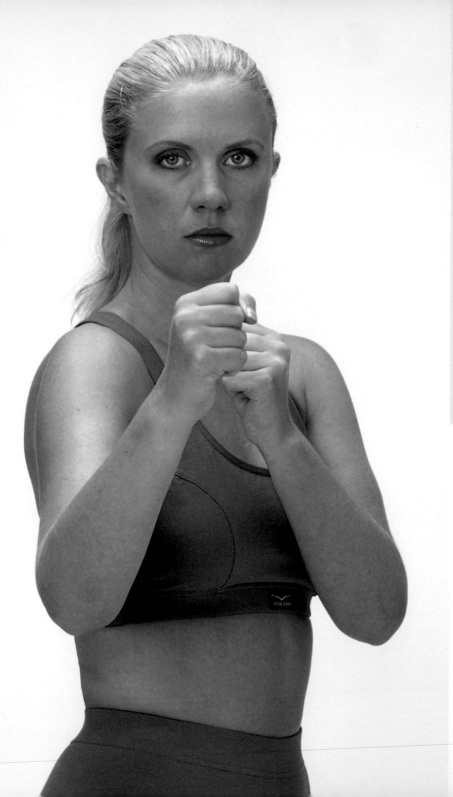

C Front hook

From fighting stance.

With the left foot leading, rotate through the ball of the left foot lifting the heel. At the same time, bring the elbow of the front arm in a head-height 90 degree angle and drive it across the line of vision using the power from your hips.

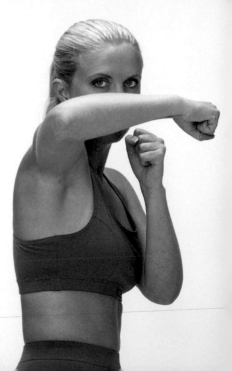

D Back hand uppercut

From fighting stance.

The uppercut begins with a hip twist bringing the back heel off the floor. The knees are bent a little more than usual in order to drive the upper cut up effectively in a vertical line. Retract quickly.

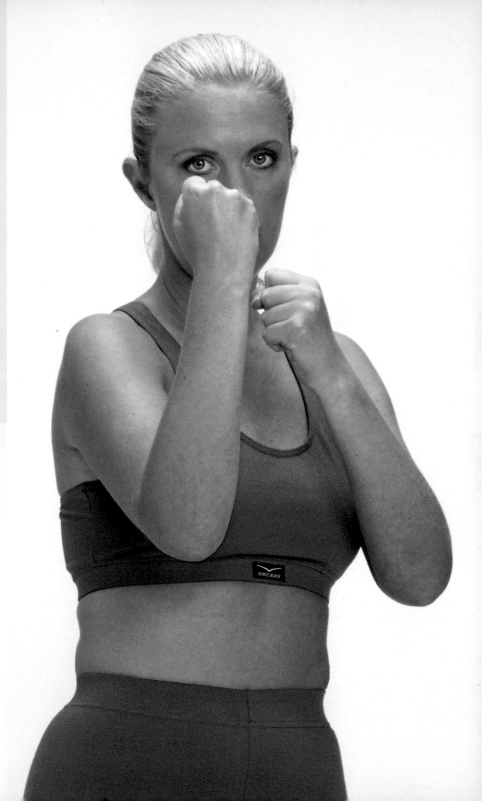

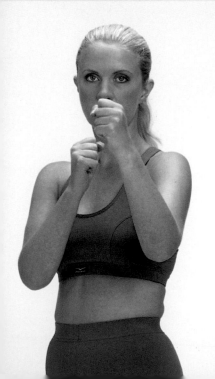

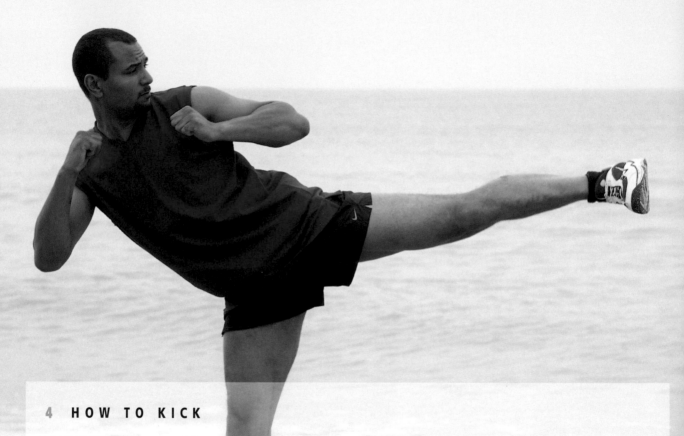

4 HOW TO KICK

For effective kicking, always visualize your imaginary target and look towards it. Never fully extend your kicking leg i.e. don't lock out your knee joints. At the same time keep your supporting leg 'soft', so again the knee joint isn't locked. Breathe out as you kick. Inhale as you retract.

Remember to kick only to where feels comfortable for you. A high kick does not work your muscles any more effectively than a low one. Concentrate on learning good technique at a low height whilst gradually increasing your flexibility. Then you can slowly build up the height of your kicks.

As you kick remember to always keep your abdominal muscles tight and firm. Don't 'slam' the kicking foot down. Retract the kicking leg, following its original path, and place the foot down in its original position. Keep your arms close to your body. Resist the temptation to throw your arms out as you are learning to balance.

Finally, remember the correct position of the foot is vital and there is a different striking point for different kicks.

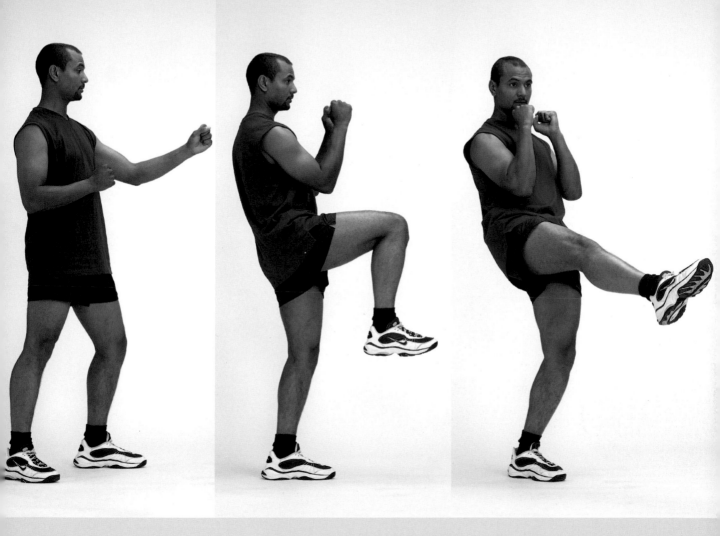

A Front kick

From fighting stance.

Bring the rear leg forward with the knee well bent and the shin vertical. Then extend this leg, letting the upper body move slightly back. The kick is delivered with the ball of the foot, with the toes pulled back. Elbows and arms are kept firm but relaxed in front of the body. Retract and place the foot down quickly without slamming!

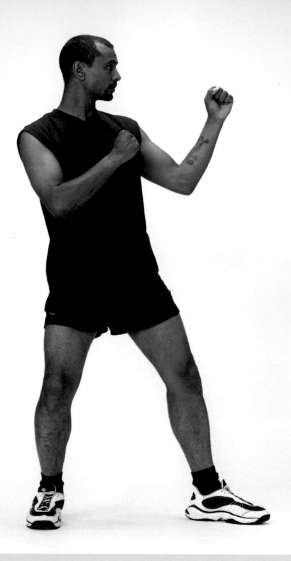
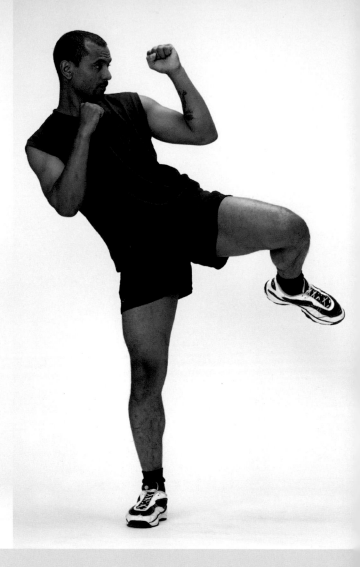

▲

B Front leg turning kick

From back stance.

The turning kick leads the foot in a horizontal curve into the target. Firstly ensure the supporting foot is turned sideways. The body weight is kept on the bent back leg. Raise the front leg up with the knee well bent. When the knee reaches hip or waist height kick out to the side (either with the instep or the ball of the foot). Use the hips to drive the kick through. Pull the kick back returning to original stance. Keep the arms and elbows up throughout kick.

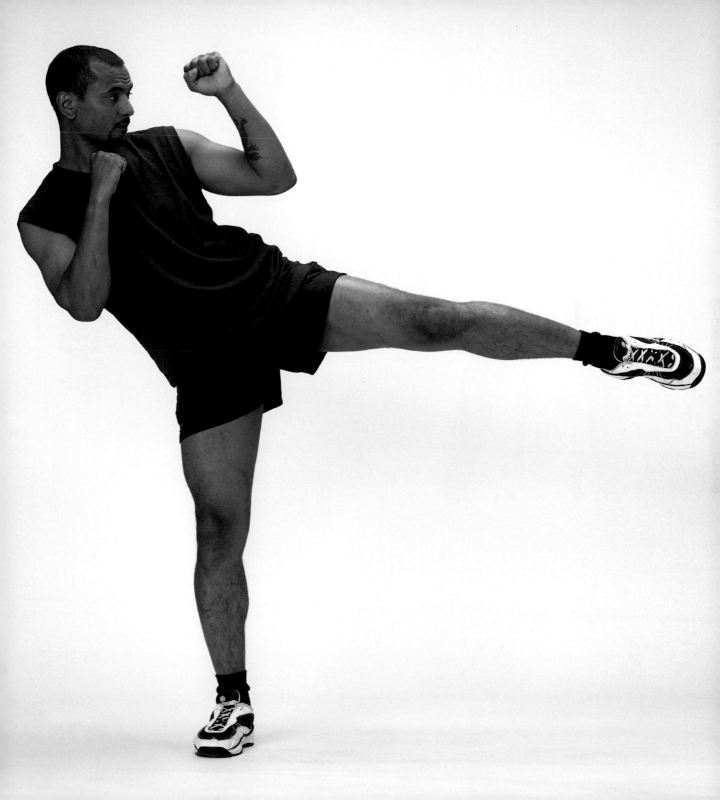

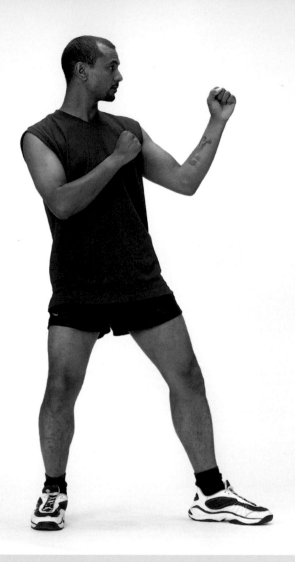
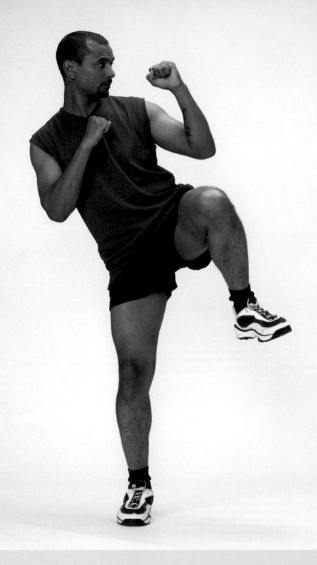

C **Front leg side kick**

From back stance.

Ensure the supporting foot is turned slightly behind and the body weight is kept on the bent back leg. Bend the front knee whilst drawing it close to the chest. Kick out the leg, keeping it in a straight line, with the toes back and aiming with the heel. Try to keep the upper body still throughout the kick. Withdraw leg taking care to bend knee before bringing it down to the floor in a controlled manner.

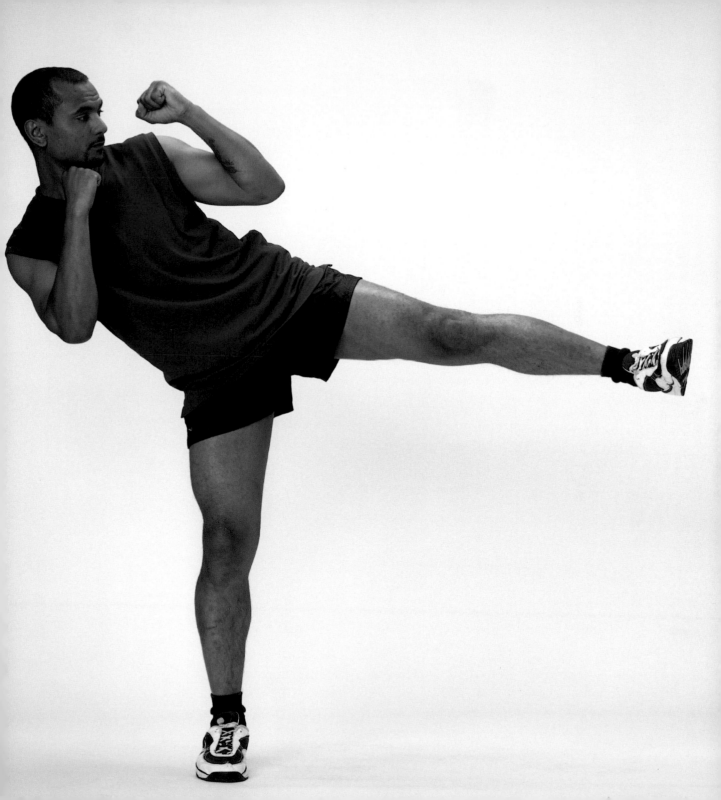

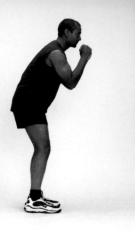
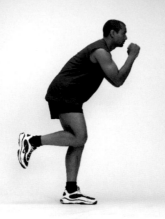

D Back kick

From back kick stance.

Lift kicking heel up towards your bottom keeping the knees close together. Your supporting weight is now on the bent leg. Leading with the heel, drive the kick behind in a straight line while at the same time rotating the head in the direction of the kick so the eyes can see the target. Kick back straight, holding your abdominal muscles tight. To withdraw do the same in reverse.

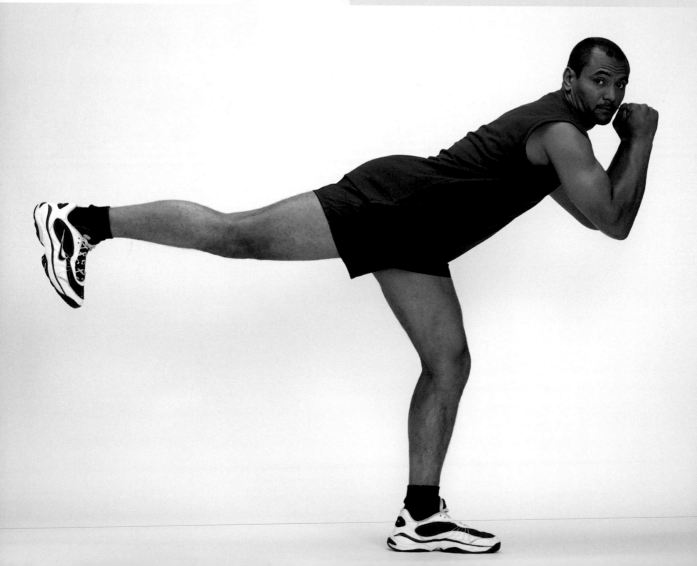

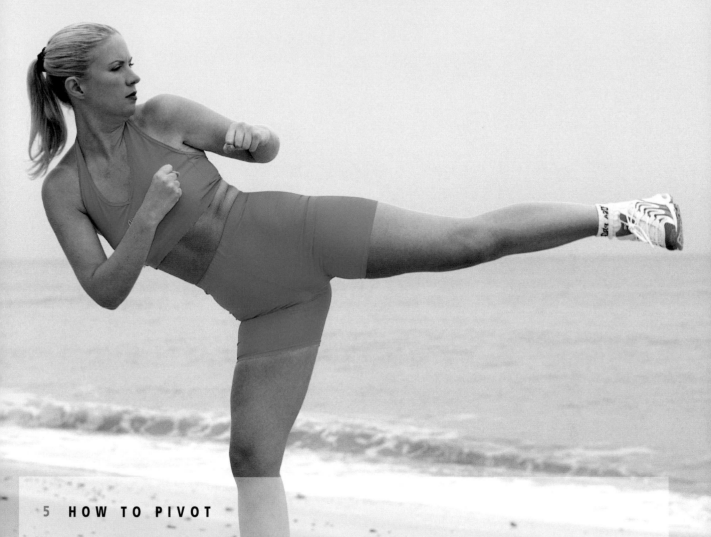

5 HOW TO PIVOT

To gain full momentum and power, your ankle must work in unison with your knees and hips. The supporting foot is a very important factor. Your supporting ankle is not only taking all of your body weight during a kick but is also maintaining your balance and acting as a part of your whole body movement. If you only pivot through the top part of your body leaving the lower half behind, many an injury can occur!

A perfect pivot

Make sure your feet are in the correct position for the stance and kick or punch. Be aware of which way your foot is going to be moving. Remember that your foot is just the base point of your pivot. Everything else is going to follow through simultaneously. Always look in the direction you are turning.

Improving balance

It does take a while and a bit of practice to improve your balance. Try the following exercises whenever you have a moment and your balance will improve surprisingly quickly!

1   Stand on your left leg, with your right leg bent and the foot placed on your right calf or thigh (depending on where feels comfortable). Hold your hands together as if you are praying. Then try it on the other side. Then try it with your eyes closed! In yoga this posture is called The Tree.

2   Use a support. Practise your kicks (and pivots) while holding onto a support. Make sure your support is stable, such as a heavy chair or a door frame. It might sound obvious but make sure whatever you use can take your weight, and is not going to either collapse or shoot away from you. Remember that the support is only there to help you with your balance. Leaning on it too hard is not only cheating (since you are not doing the kicks correctly) but you are also hindering your balance improvement.

NB. Don't get too reliant upon the support. Remember you are trying to rely on it less and less. Try letting go slowly – start from using your entire hand to just your fingers through to only a couple of fingers and then none.

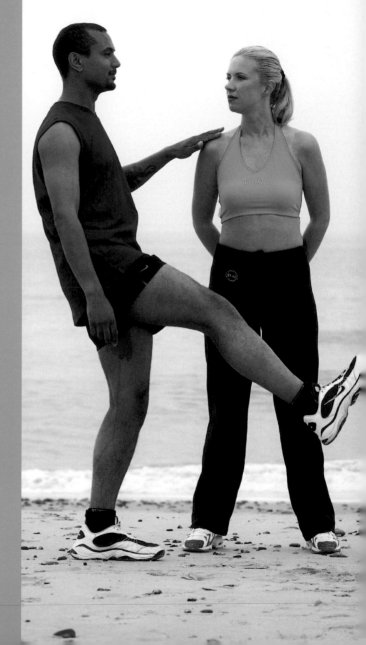

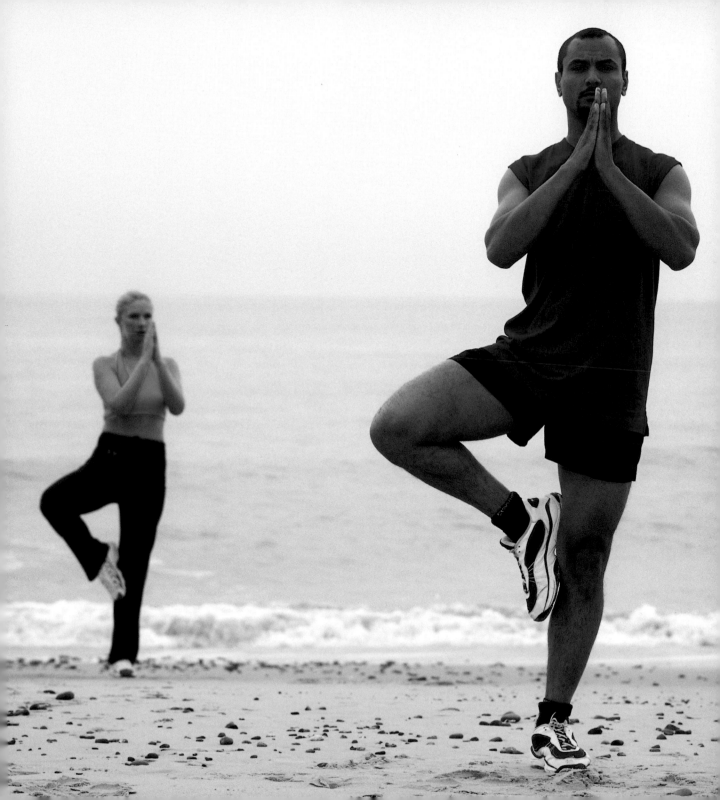

SAFE KICKING

The American Council on Exercise has compiled this list of potential risks involved in kick boxing-based exercises, with some safer alternatives:

- AVOID Overextended, far-reaching kicks.
- SAFE OPTION Omit high kicks until you are used to the routine and your flexibility has improved.
- AVOID Locking your knees, elbows and other joints when throwing punches and kicking.
- SAFE OPTION Keep all joints slightly flexed to cushion the blows.
- AVOID Pushing yourself to do more when you are feeling tired.
- SAFE OPTION Kick boxing is exhausting if you're not used to it – listen to your body and ignore anyone who urges you to do more than you feel is safe.
- AVOID Wearing or holding weights while throwing punches – this increases the risk of injury.
- SAFE OPTION Learn to do the basic moves well instead. Then try more repetitions rather than more weight.
- AVOID Repeating high-intensity exercises using the same muscle group over an extended period of time.
- SAFE OPTION Do a balanced mix of exercises for all the body.

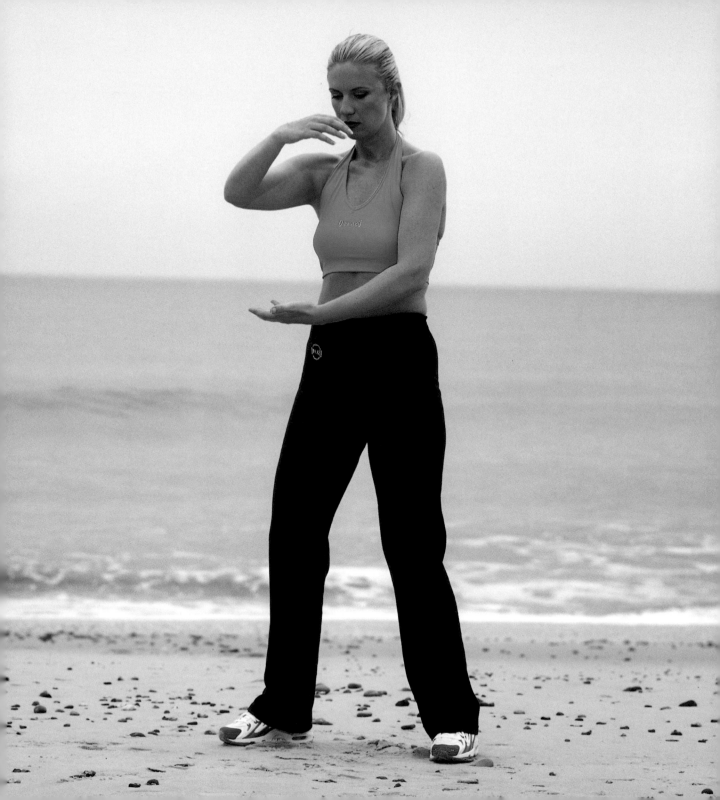

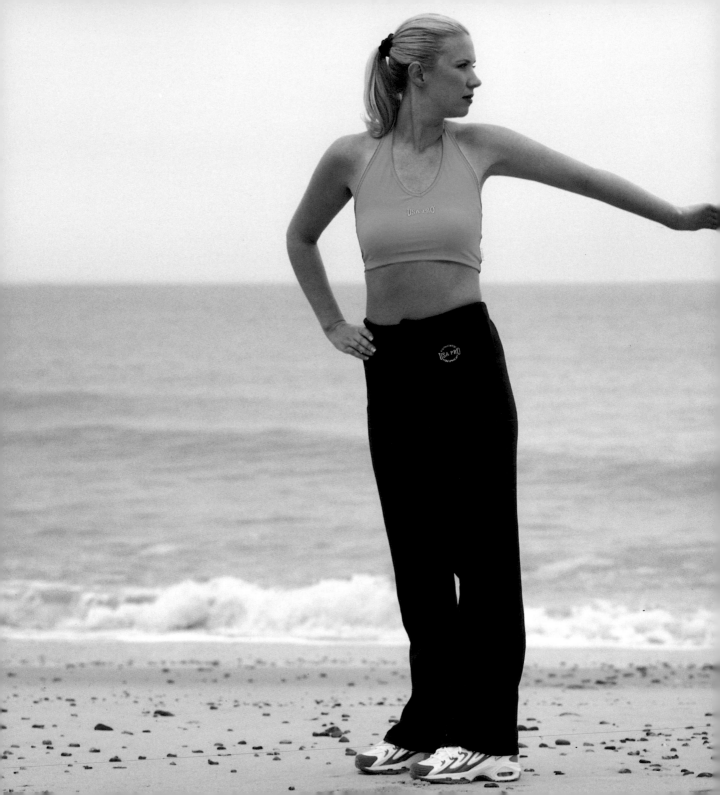

CHAPTER FOUR

WARMING UP AND COOLING DOWN

You can't read a book or magazine article about exercise without the inevitable references to the importance of warming up and cooling down. In the back of your mind, you might be thinking that it's one of those things that doesn't *really* matter, or that doesn't apply to you. It's true, that whether there is any need to stretch before *and* after a workout has been the subject of much debate in the exercise industry. But that doesn't mean it's safe to disregard this part of exercise – and here's why.

At present, the consensus is that a warm-up is essential before a workout, but not necessarily stretches, while a cool-down and stretches are both essential *after* a workout. So whether you choose to stretch before a workout is up to you, and may come down to your natural flexibility, or how you are feeling that day. The more loose-limbed among us may feel comfortable going into kicks and punches after a warm-up alone, but those who find themselves stiff and tense after a day's working at a computer, for instance, would be better advised to warm up thoroughly *and* stretch before a workout.

The warm-up serves two purposes: it prevents injuries (easier to acquire than you might think, and they can be mighty painful!), and improves your performance. It is also a time to prepare yourself not only physically, but mentally, for the workout to come. It's a way of becoming focused on your body, moving your attention from outside concerns such as work or the journey home, to what is happening inside your body, how it feels and whether there are any niggles or stiffness.

While you warm up, try to be aware of how each body part feels, and 'reconnect' with your muscles, ligaments and joints. Technically, while you are warming up you are gradually raising your heart rate. Taking the rate of activity up slowly allows the body to adapt efficiently to increase blood and oxygen flow to the heart and muscles. That will mean you are able to exercise longer, more comfortably and more efficiently than you would if you launched into a strenuous routine cold.

So it's time for a rethink. Think warm-up, and think, essential, enjoyable, useful! After your warm-up, take a short break to drink some water, take off a layer of clothing, and focus on the workout ahead.

Similarly, stopping a strenuous activity suddenly is not a good idea. When you see athletes coming over the finishing line, they invariably start walking around after a couple of seconds rather than collapsing in a heap. This is because it's easier, believe it or not, to recover from strenuous activity by doing what's called 'active recovery', i.e. doing a less strenuous activity, than by doing nothing. It is also safer for the heart – your heart is a very strong muscle but it's not a good idea to give it shocks on a regular basis!

Cooling down is also a relaxing and satisfying feeling at the end of the workout. It's a time to focus on what you have achieved and on how great you feel. End by stretching out the major muscle groups (details of how to do this follow), which will encourage the development of long, lean muscles, and help prevent stiffness the day after your workout.

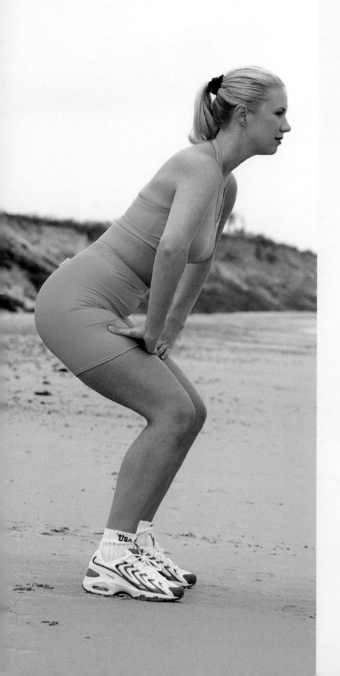

THE WARM-UP

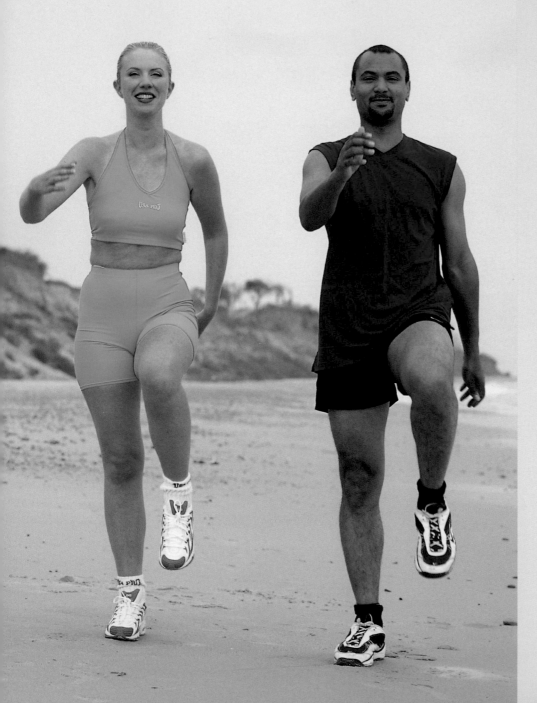

1 **March on the spot
– one minute.**

Keep your feet softly flexed
and don't 'slam' your feet
down. Always keep your back
straight and your abdominal
muscles tight. Keeping your
elbows bent, pump your arms
with your fists soft.

2 Heel digs – one minute.

Move on from a march, start placing alternate heels in front with a flexed foot. Punch your arms out straight in front with every heel dig. Keep the supporting knee soft and your back straight.

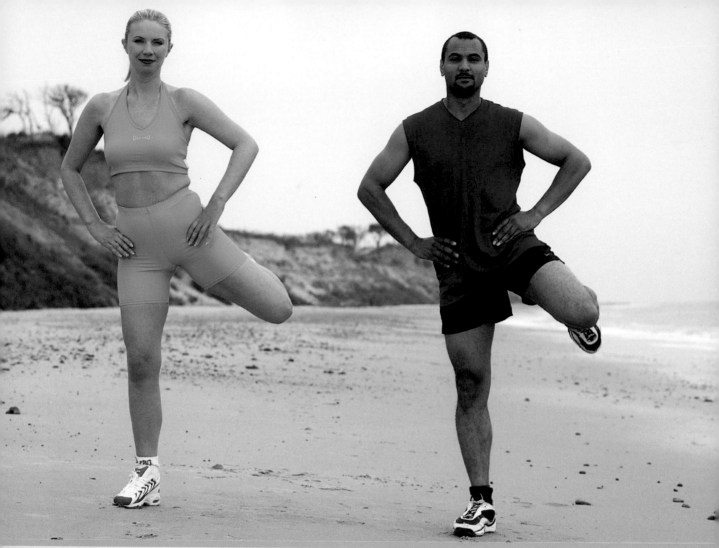

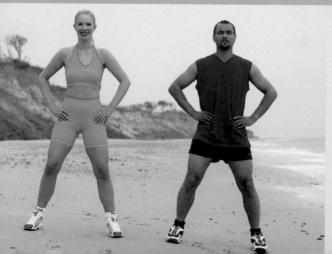

3 Leg curls – one minute.

Starting with wide legs, bring alternate heels towards your bottom. Make sure the knee of your supporting leg is again soft and your footfall is gentle. Keep your hands on your hips, punch your hands out in front or use a simple bicep curl.

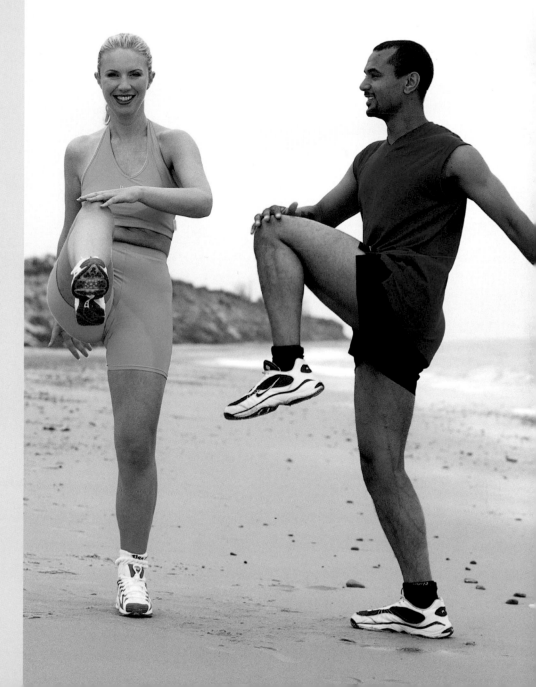

4 **Knee lifts – one minute.**

Bring one knee at a time
to the opposite hand. Don't
lean forwards or back. Keep
your abdominal muscles
tight and your back straight.
Again, make sure the knee
of your supporting leg is
not locked out i.e. slightly
soft.

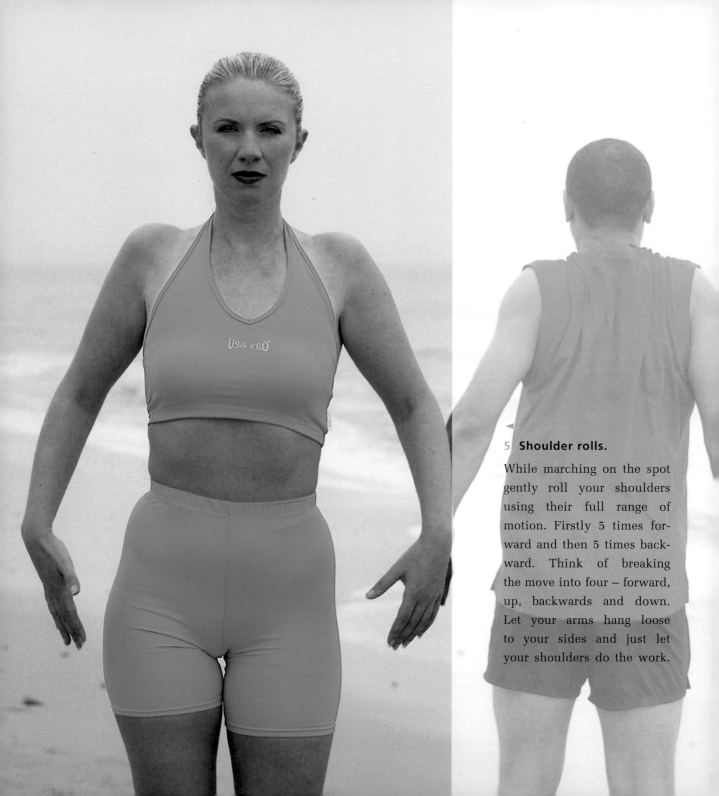

5 Shoulder rolls.

While marching on the spot gently roll your shoulders using their full range of motion. Firstly 5 times forward and then 5 times backward. Think of breaking the move into four – forward, up, backwards and down. Let your arms hang loose to your sides and just let your shoulders do the work.

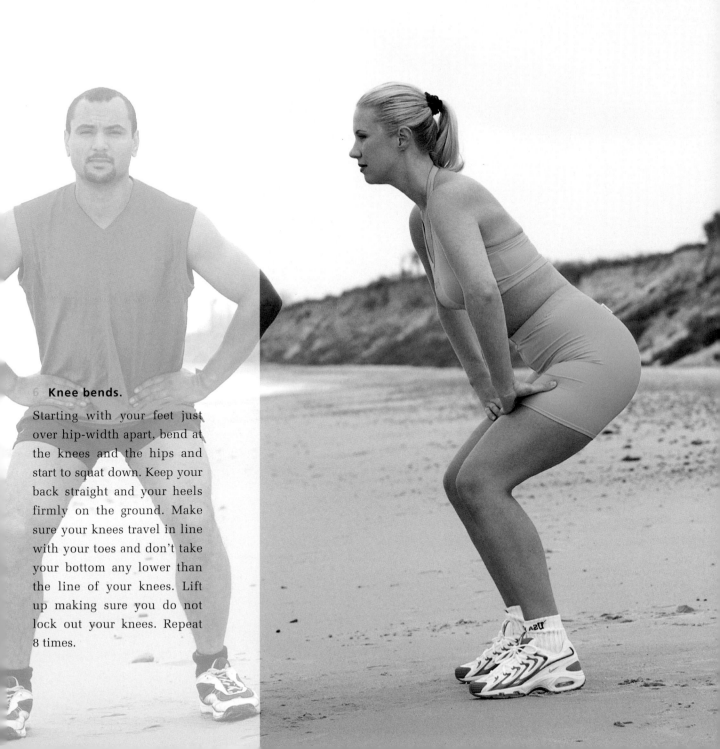

6 Knee bends.

Starting with your feet just over hip-width apart, bend at the knees and the hips and start to squat down. Keep your back straight and your heels firmly on the ground. Make sure your knees travel in line with your toes and don't take your bottom any lower than the line of your knees. Lift up making sure you do not lock out your knees. Repeat 8 times.

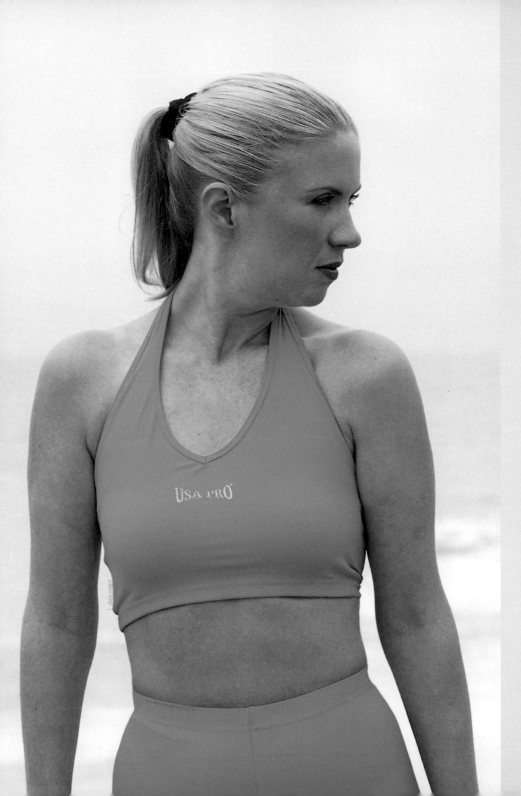

7 Neck rolls.

March gently keeping your back straight and abdominal muscles tight. Take your chin towards your right shoulder and move slowly in a semi-circle down and over to your left shoulder. Repeat from left towards right. Keep the move smooth and continuous for 8 counts.

8 Pelvic circles.

Starting with your feet hip-width apart, knees soft and back straight, place your hands above your hips and gently circle your pelvis in a 'D' shape i.e. across the back and around the front. Try to isolate the move purely to your hips, keeping your knees and upper body as still as possible. Do five times in one direction and then change and repeat other way.

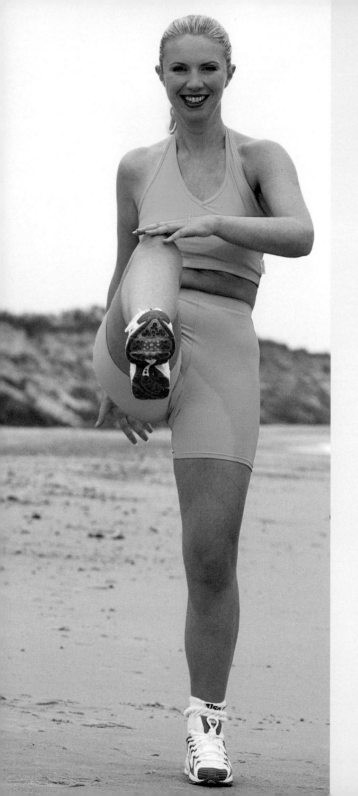

WARM-UP STRETCHES

Hold each stretch for a count of 30. You should feel pressure in a muscle, but not pain, and remember to keep breathing throughout.

1 Upper back (trapezius).

Start with your feet hip-width apart and knees slightly bent. Link the hands and reach out until you feel a stretch across the top of your back. Keep your elbows soft and chin slightly down.

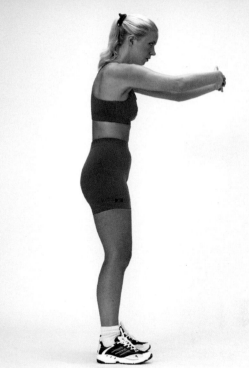

2 Back and waist (lats and obliques).

Start with your feet hip-width apart and knees slightly bent. Lean to the right and reach up with your arm. Support the torso with the opposite arm by resting the hand on the thigh. Change sides.

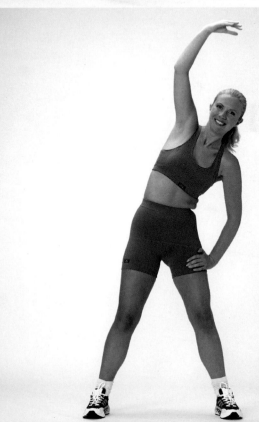

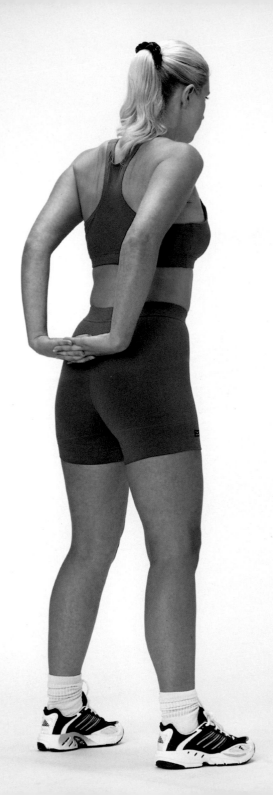

3 Chest and front of shoulders (pectorals and anterior deltoid).

Stand with the feet a little wider than hip-width apart and slightly bend the knees. Clasp the hands together behind the back and lift the hands slightly away from the body. Keep the elbows bent. You should feel the stretch across the front of the chest.

4 Front of thigh (quadriceps).

Use the wall for support if necessary. Keeping the back straight, flex the knee and grasp the ankle. Gently draw the heel to the bottom. Keep the supporting knee bent and try to keep the knees parallel. You should feel the stretch down the front of the bent thigh. Change legs.

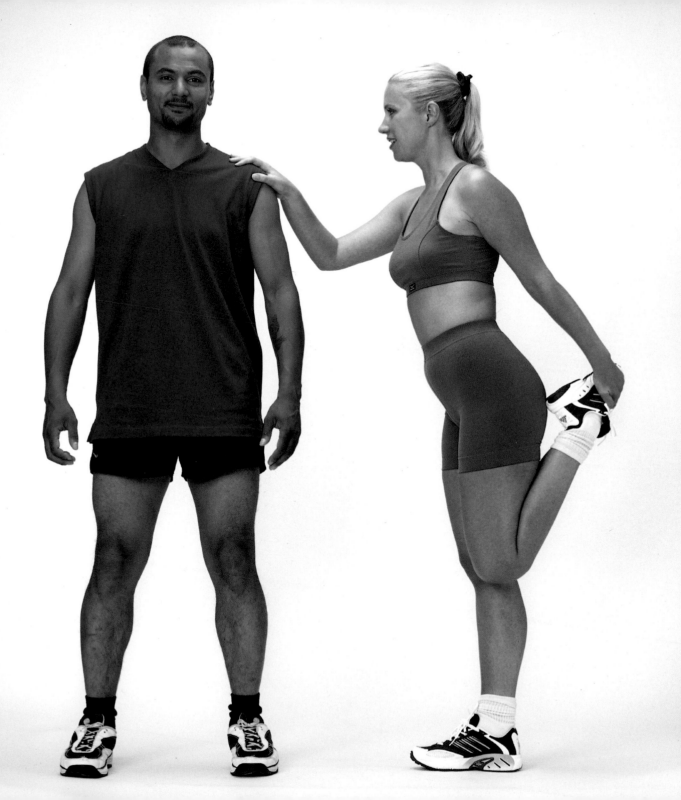

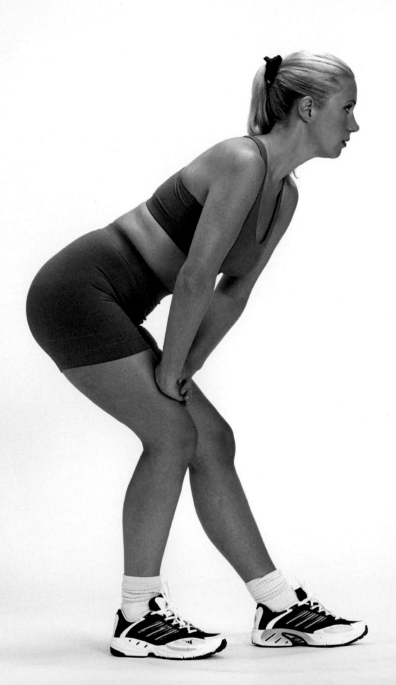

5 **Back of thigh (hamstring).**
Bend the right leg and extend the left one. Lean forwards, keeping the left leg straight but not locked. Place hands on right thigh. Aim to feel stretch in back of left thigh. Keep your back straight. Change legs.

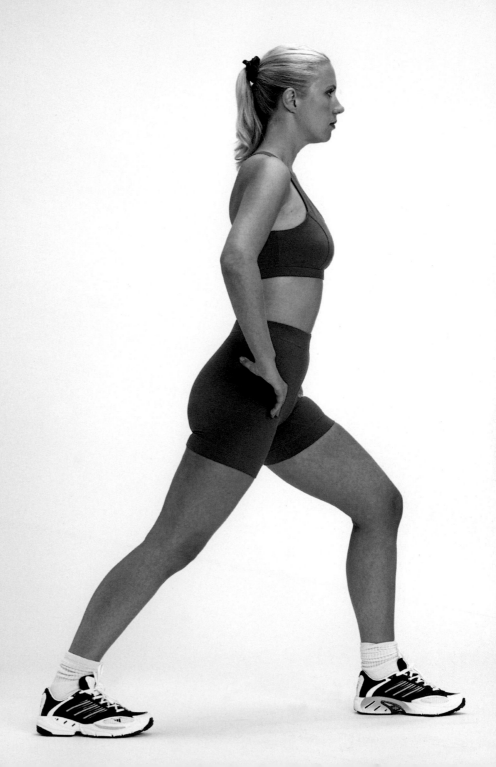

6 Calf (gastrocnemius).

Extend the right leg directly behind and bend the left front knee. Keep the hips and shoulders square and ensure the feet are hip-width apart for stability. You should feel the stretch in the upper part of the back calf. Change legs.

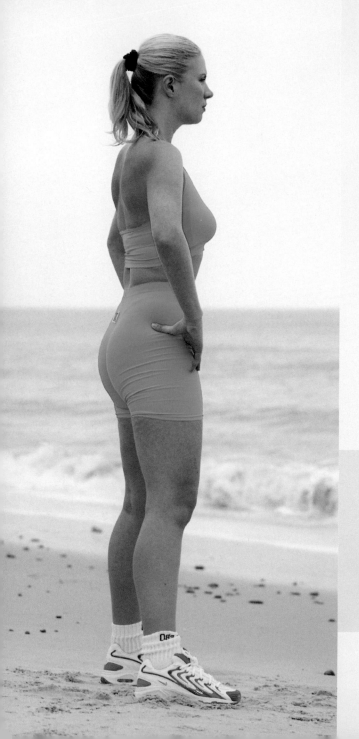

THE COOL-DOWN

Spend at least five minutes taking your heart rate down slowly and safely using exercises of decreasing intensity. Spend one minute on each of the following (in this order): front kicks, knee lifts with arms, knee lifts without arms, heel digs and marching on spot. Alternatively, simply walk around the room for five minutes, rolling your shoulders back.

Your muscles are now in prime condition to be stretched. Again, never skip this bit. If you need to shorten your workout, cut some out of the middle, rather than the beginning or the end. Stretching has many benefits ranging from injury prevention through to increasing your flexibility. It also feels great!

REMEMBER:

Hold these stretches for 30 seconds.

Stretch to a point of tension not pain!

Don't 'bounce' into the stretch. Hold them still.

Don't let yourself get cold – put a sweat top on!

Don't hold your breath. Aim for calm rhythmic breathing.

Seated hamstring stretch.

Sitting down, extend one leg in front while tucking the other one in. Keeping your back straight and your chest lifted, lean gently forwards over the straightened leg. Keep the foot flexed, toe pointing upwards and try to keep the back of the straightened leg firmly into the floor. Change legs.

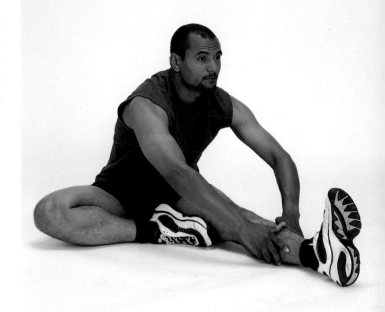

Inside thigh stretch.

Sitting up tall, draw the soles of the feet together, letting the knees drop. Hold onto your feet gently and, keeping a straight back, lean forwards. You should feel the stretch through your inner thighs.

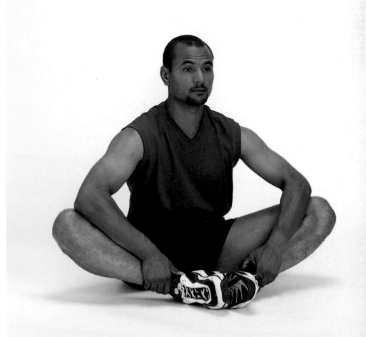

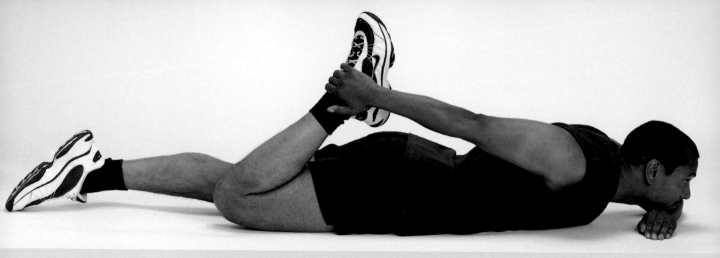

3 Front of thigh (quadriceps).

Lying on your front, rest your chin on your left hand. Reach down and grasp your right ankle with your right hand. Draw your heel towards your bottom, keeping your hips on the floor. Feel the stretch along the front of the bent thigh. Change legs.

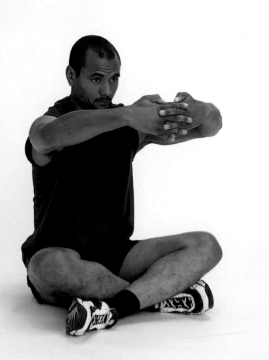

4 Upper back (trapezius).

Sit comfortably with your legs crossed. Stretch your arms out in front and interlink your fingers. Keep a bend in the elbows and drop your chin slightly. Feel the stretch across the back of the shoulders.

Back (latissimus dorsi).

From the last position, lift the arms up above the head keeping the bend in the elbows. Feel the ribcage 'lift' out of your hips. Hold.

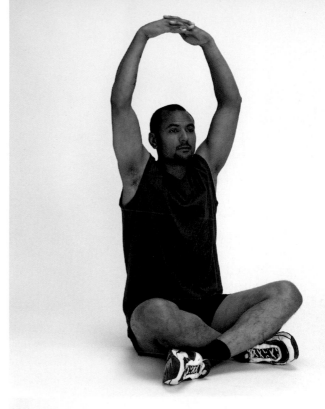

Chest and front of shoulders (pectorals and anterior deltoid).

Still sitting, take the hands behind the back and link the fingers. Keeping the elbows bent, slowly take the hands away from your bottom, feeling your shoulder blades squeeze together. Relax the chin down slightly.

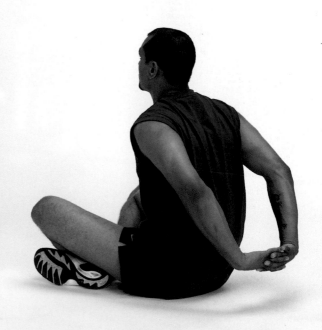

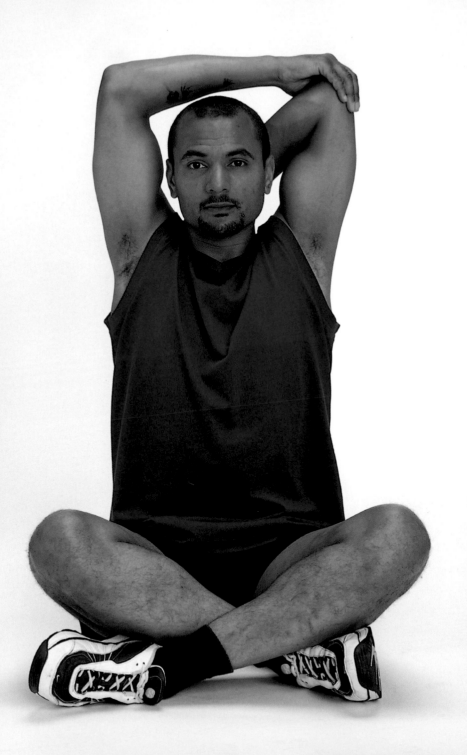

7 Back of arms (triceps).

Take the left hand up in the air and place it palm down behind your neck. Gently support with right arm, feeling the stretch along the back of the arm. Change arms.

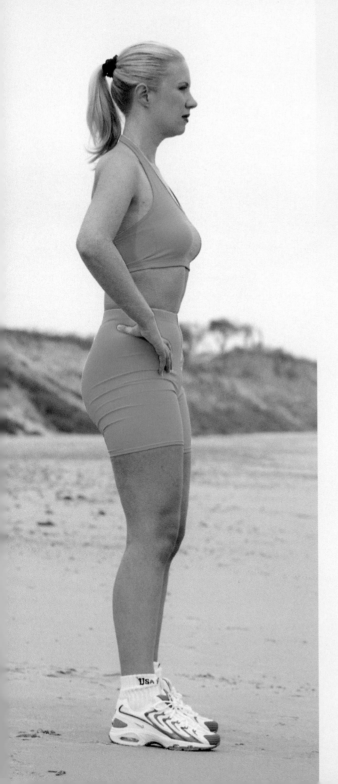

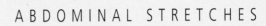

ABDOMINAL STRETCHES

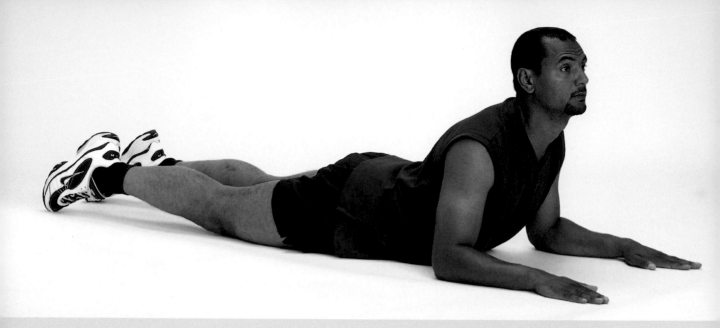

1   Lying face down on the floor, place both hands out 'sphinx'-like in front of your body. Lift chin and upper chest up and gently pull forwards using your hands. Keep the whole of your forearm flat on the floor. You should feel a gentle stretch through your abdominal region. Hold for about 15 seconds.

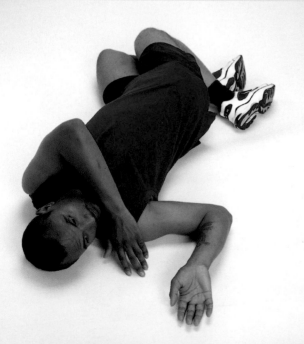

2   Lie on your back with your legs bent at the knees and your feet on the floor. Let your legs fall over to your right side, while your arms fall to the left. Hold for 30 seconds and change sides.

3   From a seated, cross-legged position, allow the upper body to slump forward over the legs. You should feel a slight tension in the lower back. Extend the back further by walking the fingers out in front as far as comfort allows.

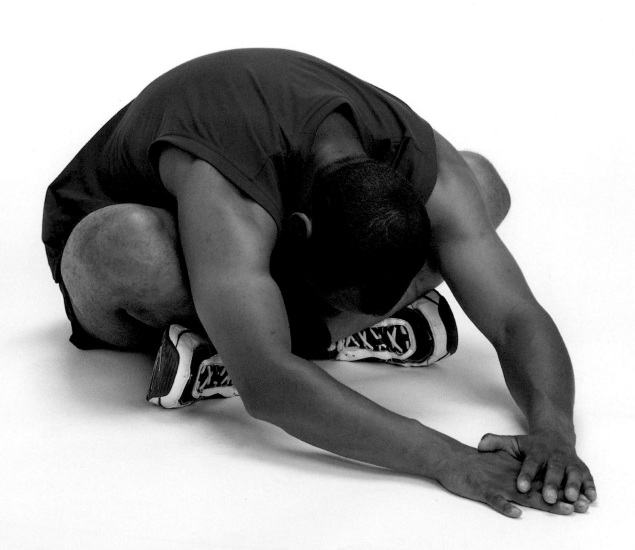

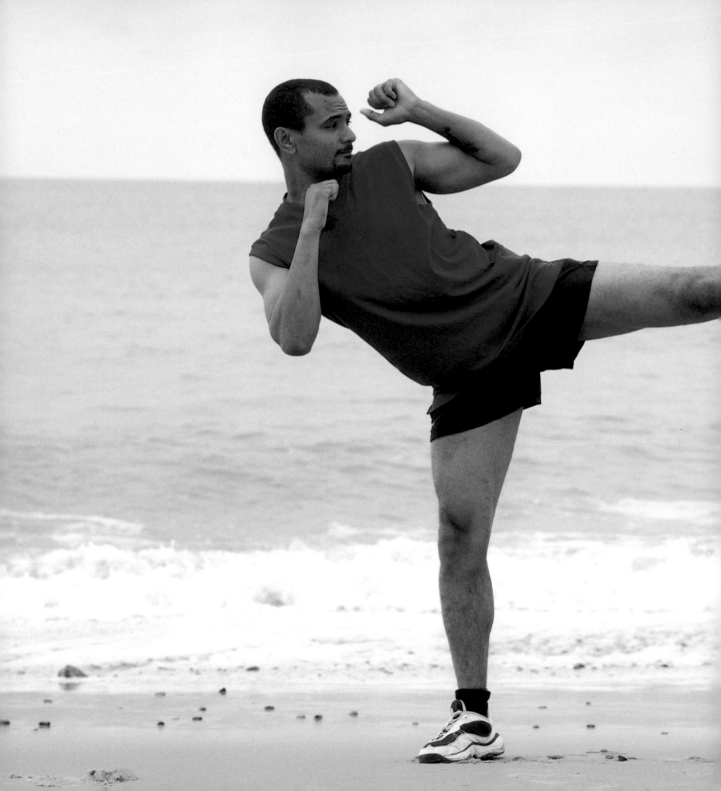

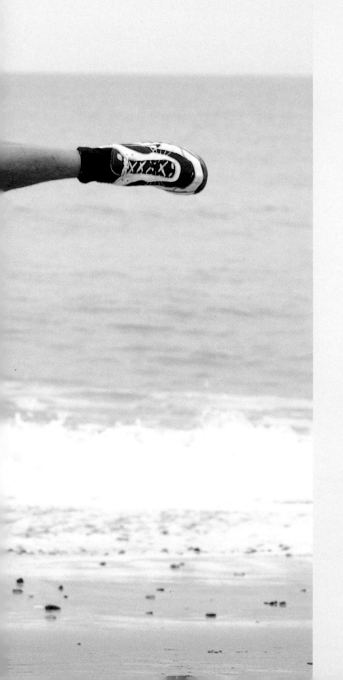

CHAPTER FIVE

LOWER BODY
WORKOUT

For many people, women in particular, the lower body is the most difficult to keep fat-free and firm. It's also the area that women are most eager to work on; let's face it, who doesn't want a pair of sleek, well-conditioned legs and a firm behind? When it comes to the legs, we usually want to target three areas in particular: that bit between the buttocks and the back of the leg, the front thigh and the inner knee. Are any of these areas your personal least-favourite body parts? Thought so!

Well, firstly, of course, I'm going to tell you to stop hating your thighs or knees and start seeing them as an integral part of your body. But secondly, I'm going to tell you how to get them into shape. The buttocks, meanwhile, are a different story. Unless you've been blessed with a naturally firm, and tight butt, after a while (particularly if you live a sedentary life) gravity takes its toll and your bottom can head South. Catch sight of it in a changing room mirror and you're likely to give it some abuse in your head. Well, next time you feel like doing that, consider that your buttocks, whatever they may look like, enable you to stand up, sit down, walk upstairs, sprint and jump. You would be lost without your buttocks. So stop cursing them, and give them a bit of attention instead.

A bonus of working the muscle groups described below, which are the largest muscle groups of your body, is that as well as toning you up, you are boosting your metabolic rate and burning off fat at the same time. So here's what you'll be working:

Gluteus maximus – Namely your butt (this also includes the lesser known gluteus medius and minimus). Not only is it the biggest muscle you have, it is also the strongest.

Hamstrings – These are actually three muscles that run up the back of your leg from the knee to the hip. Since they control how your knee bends, they are key to correct kicking.

Quadriceps – The front of your thighs. Well, actually, the front, inner and outer side of each thigh. These are four powerful muscles – one links your knee to your pelvis; the other three run from the knee area up along the thighbone. Again, they are important kicking muscles allowing you to extend your leg.

Adductors and abductors – Inside and outside thigh muscles (much easier terms to remember). The outside thigh muscle (abductors) help lift and move your leg away from your body while the inside thigh muscle (adductors) helps bring your leg back towards your body.

Gastrocnemius and soleus – Calf muscles, not thought about often but imperative to movement. Gastrocnemius is your upper calf muscle while soleus is the lower one. Every time you point and flex those toes, those muscles work.

Hip flexors – Not quite lower body but highly important. Flexors are muscles that flex joints – hip flexors help raise the leg in your knee lifts and kicks.

The general aim of this workout is to tighten and lift your butt, tone and strengthen your hamstrings and define and tighten those quadriceps. As you can see, the lower body is made up of some meaty muscle groups which are already quite strong through everyday use. All of the lower body muscle groups are involved in our workout, some more than others. By combining basic resistance exercises, such as the squats, with the dynamism of the powerful kicks, we have created a highly effective lower body toner.

HOW OFTEN SHOULD I DO THIS WORKOUT?

Firstly, it is important to know that what you do is as important as what you don't do. There is no point in doing the same workout day in and day out. Recovery and rest of those muscles used is as important as the workout itself. So three times a week, on alternate days, is perfect. Use the intermediate days on the upper body or ab workout.

WHEN CAN I MAKE IT HARDER?

As long as you are working out on a regular basis, then you will improve at a steady pace. Once you feel you are completing the workout with ease, it is time to increase your level. However, remember if for any particular reason you have time off exercising, go back to the original workout for a few sessions. This will help you prevent muscle soreness and injury – muscles do forget!

HOW DO I MAKE IT HARDER?

- Increase the repetitions of the squats and kicks.
- Kick a bit higher.
- Don't let the kicking foot come down between reps.
- Add some resistance to the squats by holding dumbbells.

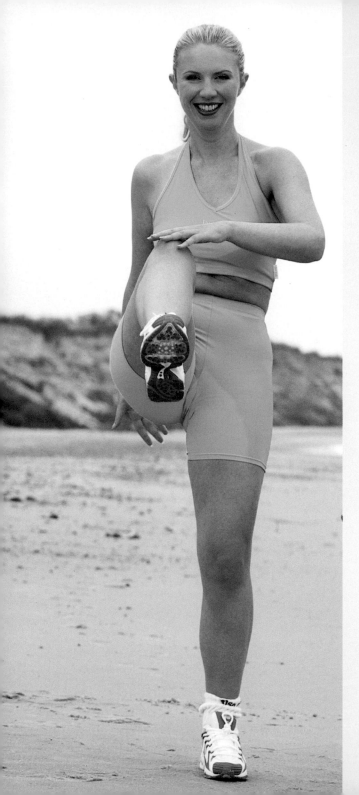

THE WORKOUT

Start with the warm-up (see page 57). Then follow the workout in this order: for instructions for individual moves, see previous chapters (although, of course, if you have mastered the basics, you don't need them).

- Basic squats x 20
- Active rest – calf raises with buttock squeeze (see over)
- Turning kick off front right leg x 15/20
- Basic squats x 20
- Turning kick off front left leg x 15/20
- Active rest
- Right leg back kick left x 20
- Left leg front kick x 20
- Left leg back kick x 20
- Right leg front kick x 20
- Squat – side kick to right – squat – side kick to left x 20
- Active rest
- Left knee x 20
- Right front kick x 20
- Right side kick x 20
- Right back kick x 20
- Right knee x 20
- Active rest
- Left front kick x 20
- Left side kick x 20
- Left back kick x 20
- Cool down and stretches

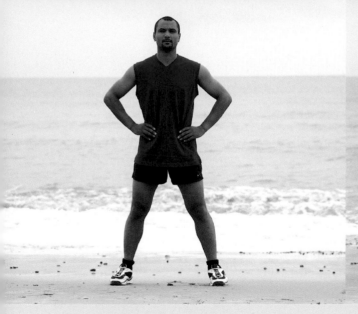

Basic squats

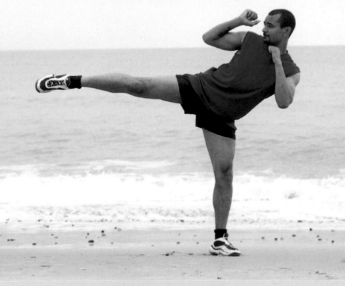

Turning kick off front right leg

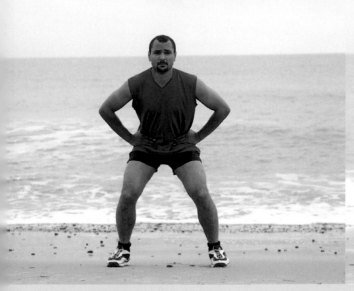

Basic squats

Turning kick off front left leg

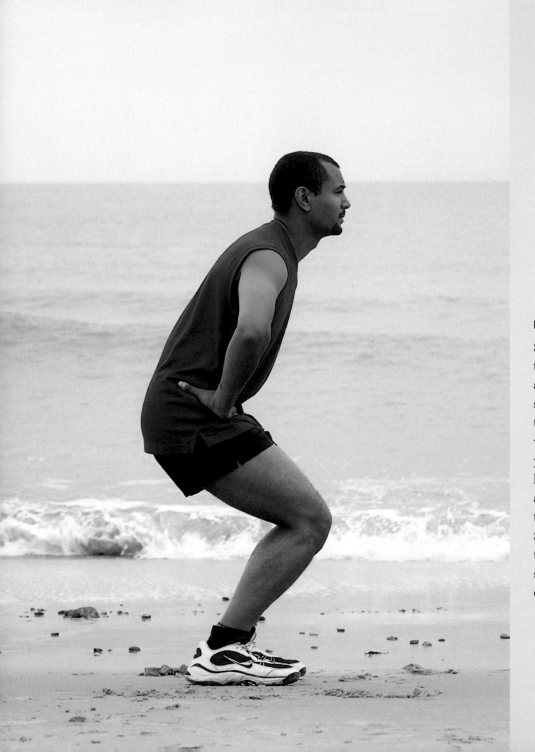

Basic squat

Stand with feet one and a half times hip-width apart. Flexing at the knees and the hips, squat to a position where the thighs are roughly parallel with the ground. Do not take your bottom lower than your knees. Keep your back flat and your abdominal muscles tight throughout the move. Straighten up, taking care not to lock out your knees. Make sure your knees do not go over your toes.

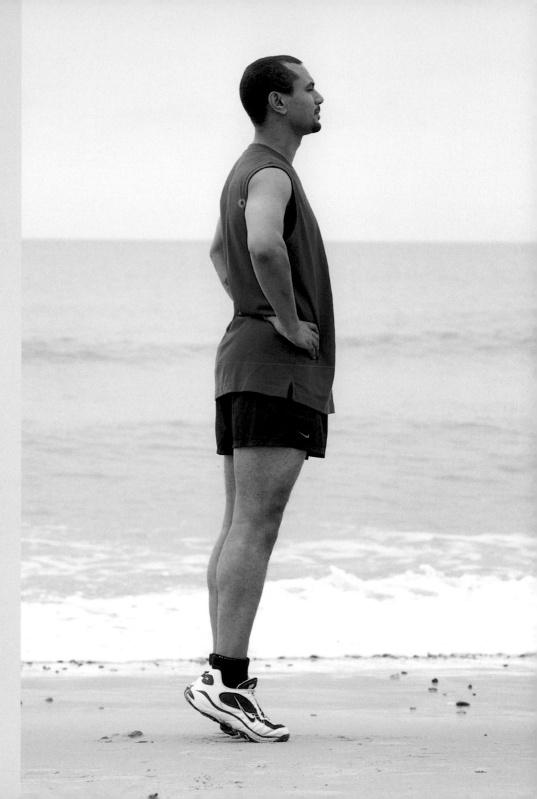

Active rest – Calf raises with buttock squeeze

Keeping the feet hip-width apart and knees soft, rise up onto the balls of your feet taking care to keep weight even over each foot. Squeeze your buttocks when you reach the highest point and return gently to ground. Resist the urge to rock back on your heels when you land – think that you are just 'touching' the floor before lifting up again straight away.

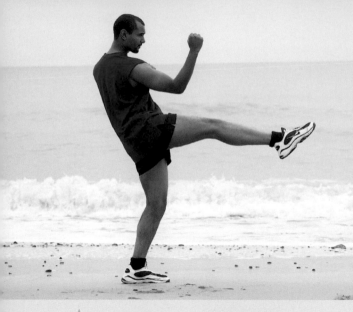
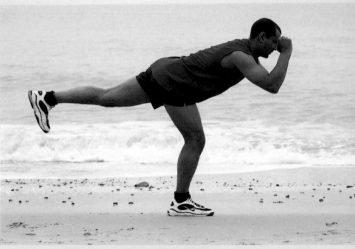

Right leg back kick – left leg front kick x 20

Right leg back kick – left leg front kick x 20

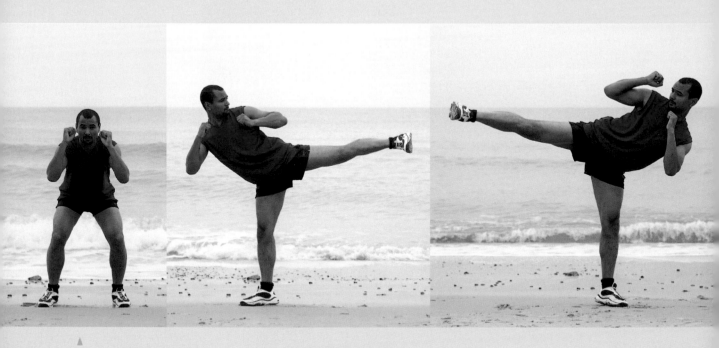

Squat – side kick to left – squat – side kick to right x 20

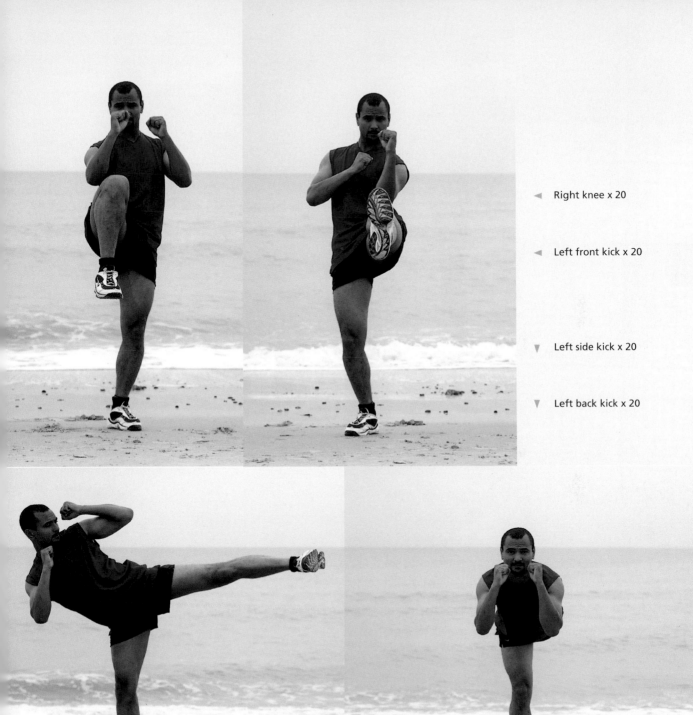

Right knee x 20

Left front kick x 20

Left side kick x 20

Left back kick x 20

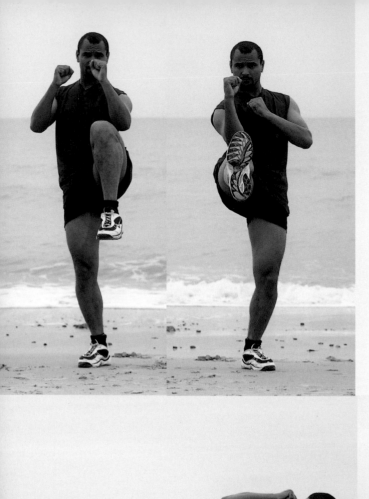

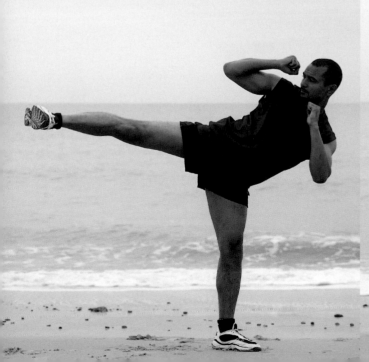

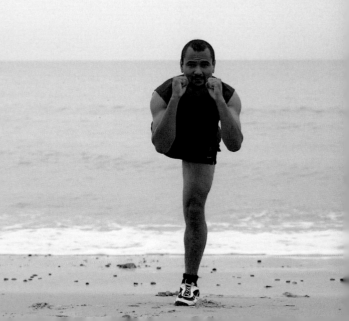

◄ Left knee x 20

◄ Right front kick x 20

▼ Right side kick x 20

▼ Right back kick x 20

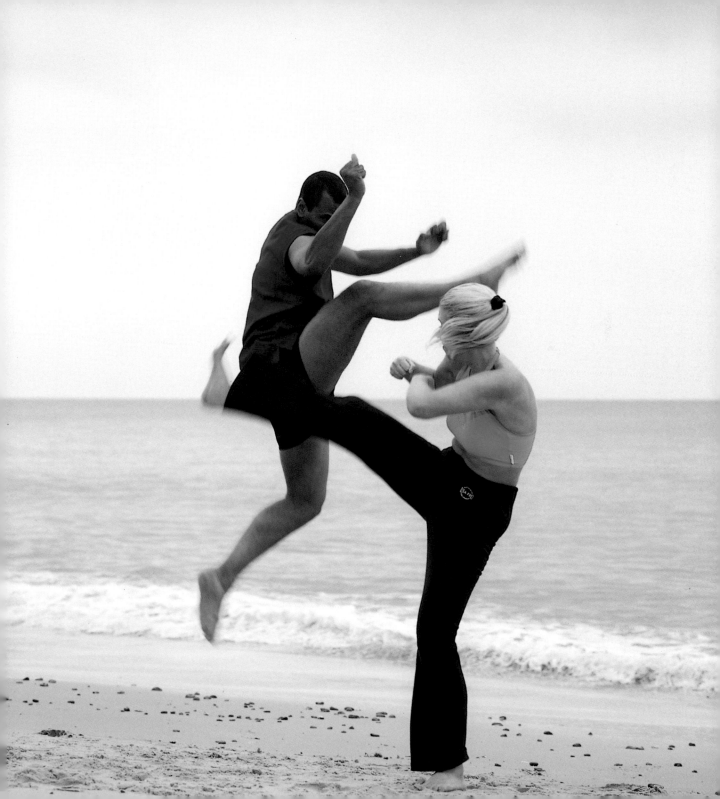

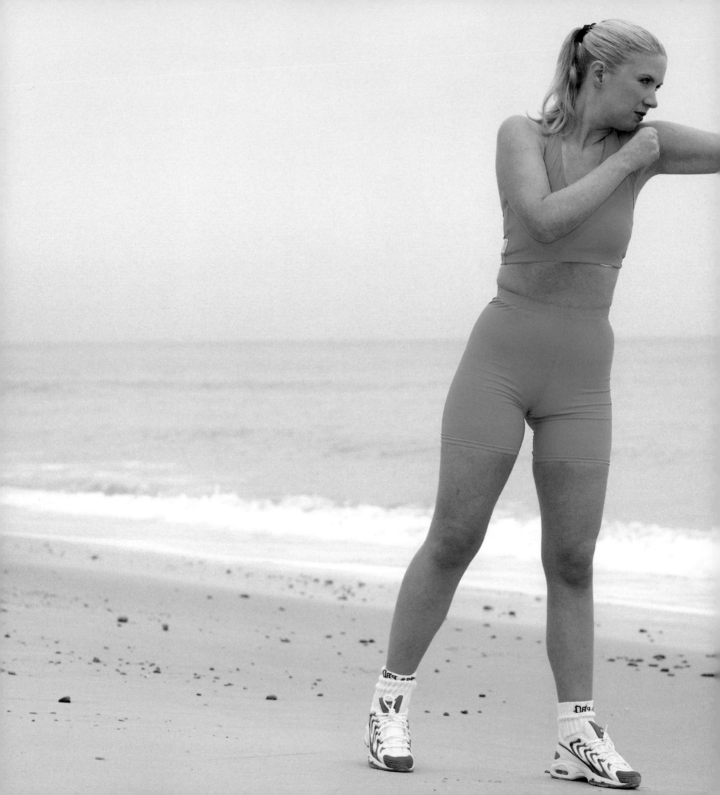

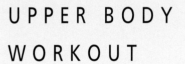

CHAPTER SIX

UPPER BODY WORKOUT

Why train the upper body? If you're male, you won't need an answer to this question. If you're female, you probably will. The answer is that upper body training imparts a graceful appearance to your arms and shoulders, and provides extra power for everyday activities such as lifting and pushing. It can also help you balance out a pear shape (a larger bottom half is less noticeable if your upper half is toned and shapely). And if you care about being trendy, you'll know that defined arms are *de rigeur* with your vest top and combat trousers (*a la* All Saints and Madonna).

The exercises in this routine require integrated movement, recruiting the muscles in your chest and shoulders as well as your arms. It also pays attention to the triceps which are very hard to target – and the reason why so many women have those saggy underarms they hate! Here's exactly what you'll be working:

- **Pectorals** ('pecs' for short) – The main muscle in your chest. These are pushing muscles which is why press-ups and dips are great individual workouts for this muscle group. Pectoralis major (there is also a minor) is the muscle that delivers your punch!
- **Latissimus dorsi and trapezius** – Namely your back muscles (this does also include your lower back muscle but we are dealing with that in your abdominal workout). Your 'lats' form a large triangle across your back, from under your armpit, along most of your spine, ending below your waist. You work your lats every time you move your arm back or up and mainly in this workout, when you recover your punch. Trapezius (or 'traps' from now on) is another triangle shaped muscle that comes from your lower neck to the middle of your back. It helps you with your posture, keeps your upper body erect and helps you lift your arms.
- **Deltoids** – Shoulder muscles. These run like shoulder pads over your shoulders. They assist you in moving your arms up, down, forward and back.
- **Biceps and triceps** – Namely front and back of arm muscles. Poor triceps are the cause of many a saggy arm! It is a pushing muscle and works in this case when you deliver a punch. It also works it conjunction with your pecs when you do a dip or a press-up. Your biceps do the opposite work – it is a pulling muscle. Again, it works when you punch.

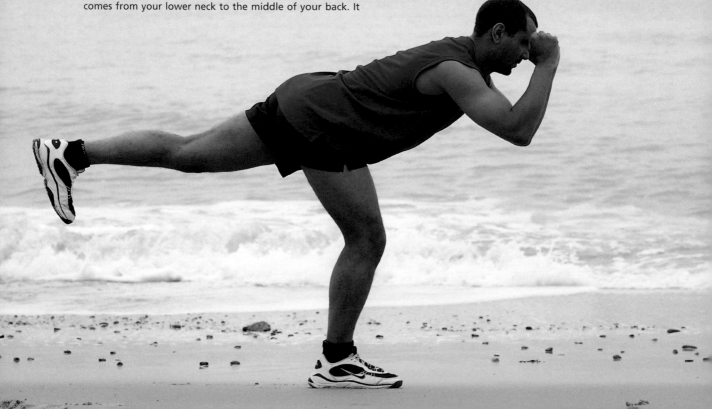

HOW OFTEN SHOULD I WORK MY UPPER BODY?

The same principles apply to all workouts – namely recovery is as important as the workout itself. Give your upper body muscles adequate rest before you work them again. Try doing this workout on alternate days.

WHEN CAN I MAKE IT HARDER?

When you can flow through the exercises with ease – you will know the next day if the workout has had any effect. You should never feel in any pain, but a slight tension within the muscle group worked is an indicator of a good workout. Remember though, pain is not good!! This means you have damaged yourself, which is not the intention at all.

HOW DO I MAKE IT HARDER?

- Do your punches twice as fast – using perfect technique.
- Add more repetitions.
- Combine the above.
- Increase the resistance on your tricep dips.

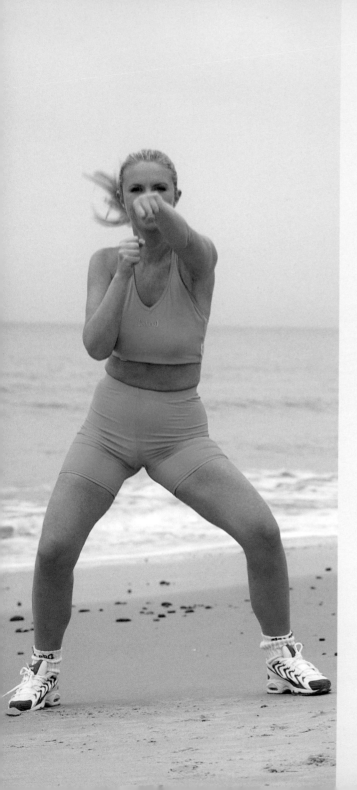

THE WORKOUT

- Warm-up
- Basic stance with hands up. Punch left/right x 20 each side
- Lateral raise x 20
- Triceps dips x 15
- Active rest – 15 power jumps
- Repeat punches
- Repeat lateral raise
- Active rest – 15 power jumps
- Basic stance punches
- Pec decks x 20
- Wall press-ups x 15
- Half press-ups x 10
- Active rest – 15 power jumps
- Basic stance punches
- Wall press-ups x 15
- Basic stance punches
- Active rest
- Standing flyes x 20
- Cool-down

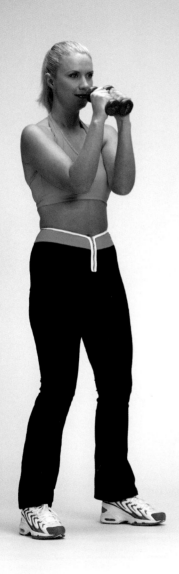

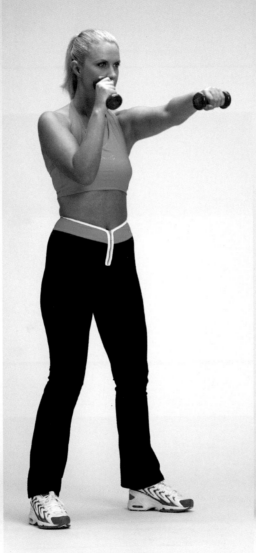

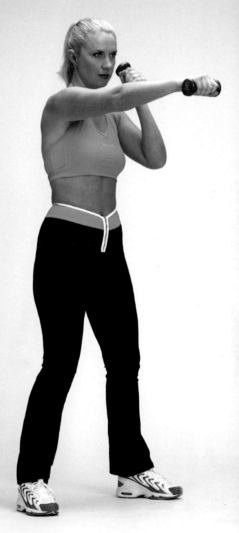

Basic stance with hands up.

Punch left.

Punch right.

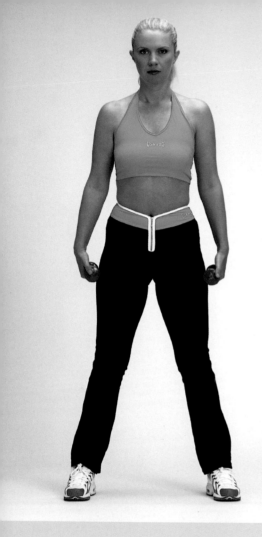 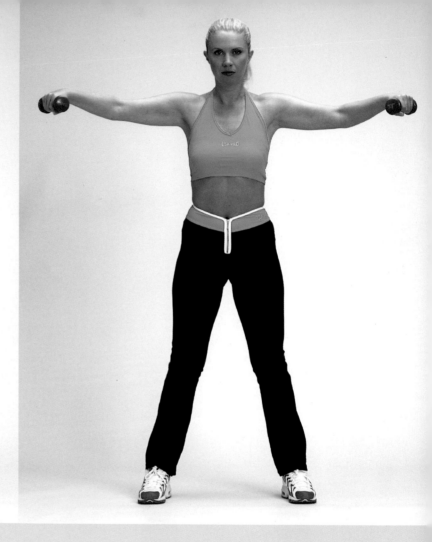

Lateral raise x 20

Lateral raise

Keeping a slight bend in your elbows raise your hands to shoulder height keeping your palms facing down. Return to start position slowly.

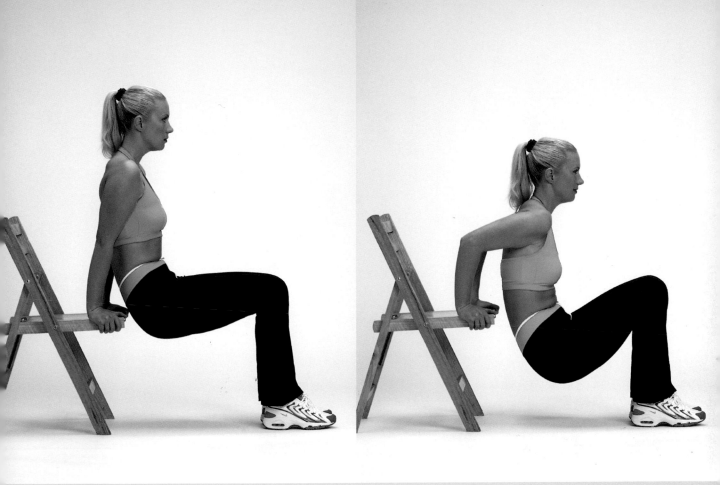

Triceps dips x 15

Triceps dips

Firstly it is very important to use something stable for this exercise! Place your hands either side of your body holding on gently to your support. Keeping your back straight and your abdominal muscles tight, lower your butt gently, bend at the elbows. Keep your back close to your support and do not take your elbow angle past 45 degrees.

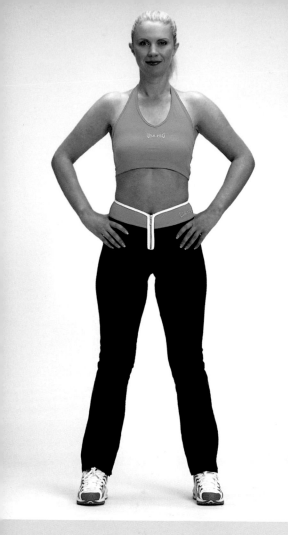
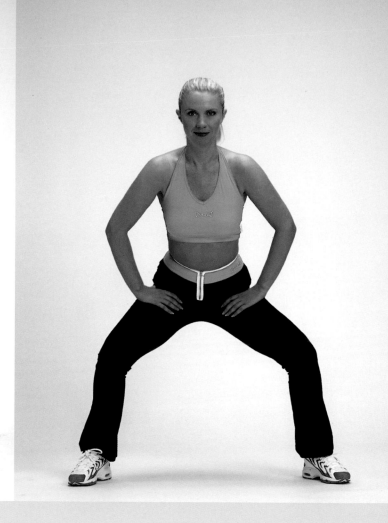

Active rest – 15 power jumps

Stand with your feet shoulder-width apart, knees soft, hands on hips. Bend at the knees and jump, taking legs out to two-and-a-half times shoulder-width apart. Return to the start and repeat.

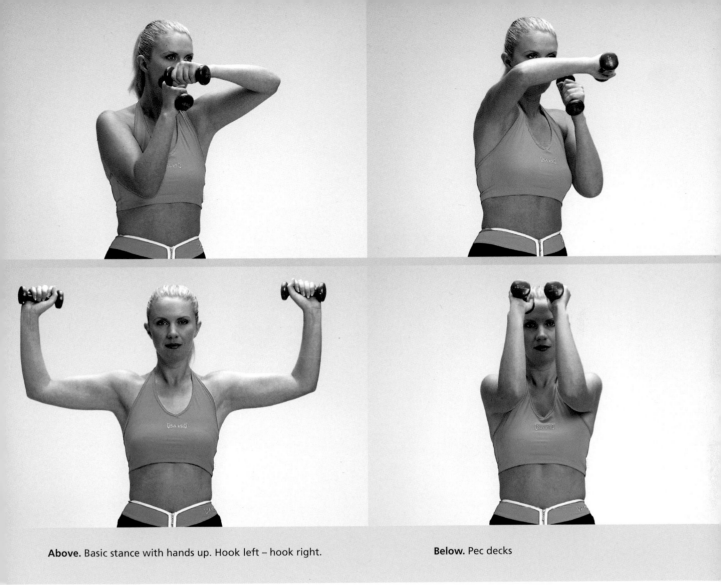

Above. Basic stance with hands up. Hook left – hook right.

Below. Pec decks

Pec-decks

Take arms out at right angles to body and then squeeze forearms together, making sure elbows and wrists touch. Keep arms high.

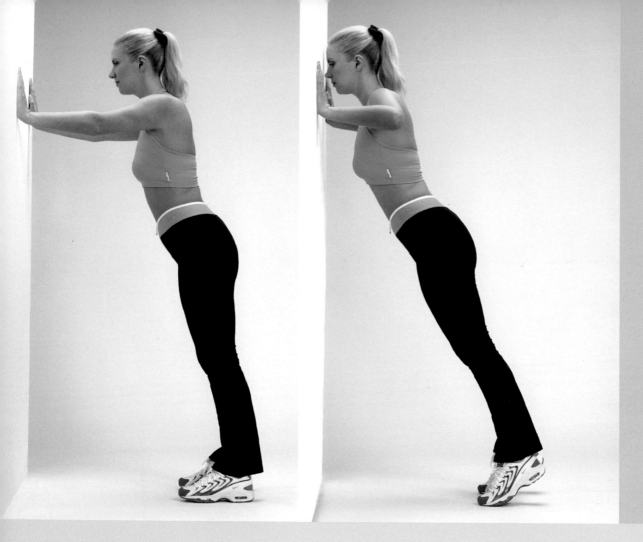

Wall press-ups x 15

Wall press-ups

Taking your hands one-and-a-half times shoulder-width apart, place them at shoulder height onto the wall. Keeping your back straight walk your legs back until you feel your body weight on your hands.

Keeping your wrists firm, bent at the elbows, lean your body towards the wall. Keep your elbows high. Straighten back up and take care not to lock out your elbows.

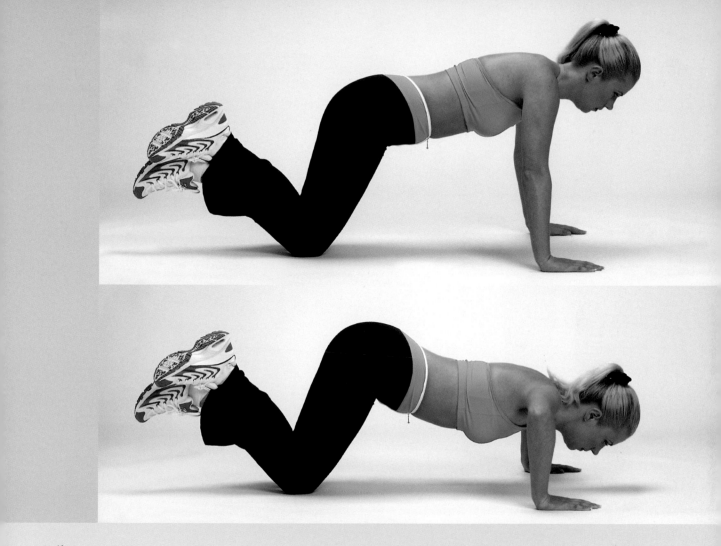

Half press-ups x 10

Half press-ups

Begin on your hands and knees, with your hands under your shoulders, taking your body weight on your hands. Lower your body to 4 inches off the floor, and push back up, using the muscles of your arms and chest. Keep your abdominals tight throughout.

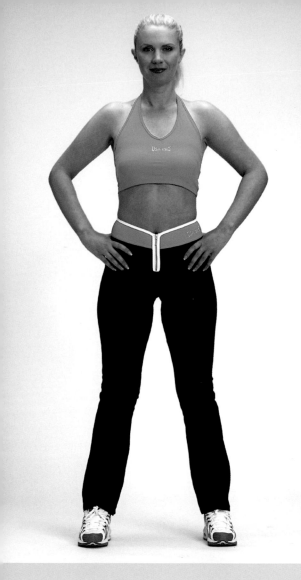

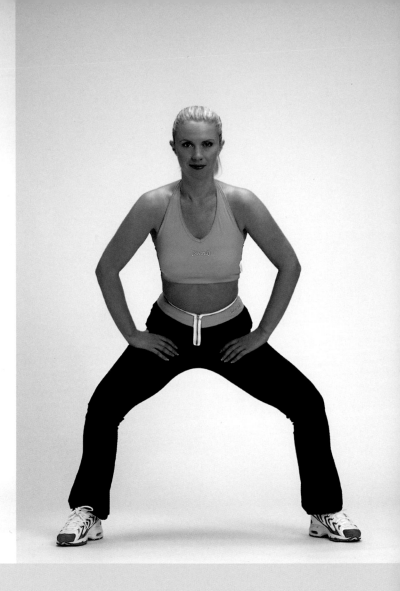

Active rest – 15 power jumps

Stand with your feet shoulder-width apart, knees soft, hands on hips, bend at the knees and jump, taking legs out to two-and-half times shoulder-width apart, bending your knees as you jump. Return to the start and repeat.

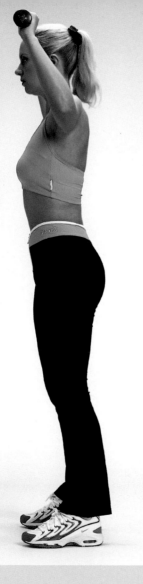
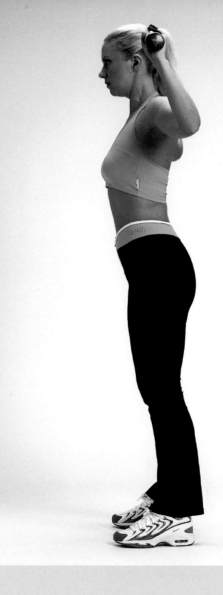

Standing flyes x 20

Standing flyes

Take arms out at right angles to body and squeeze shoulder blades together while opening up the chest. Keep arms high and visualize working the top part of your back.

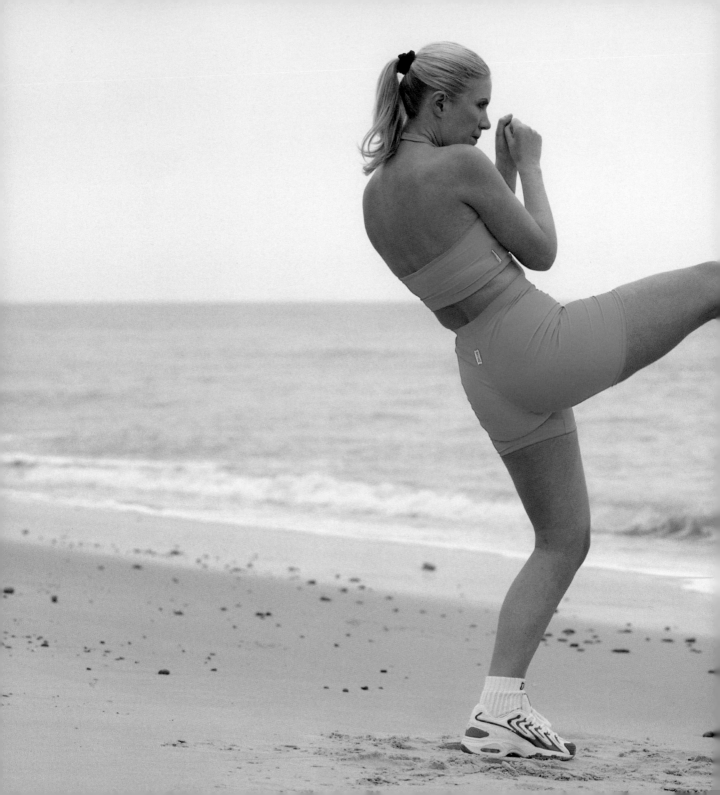

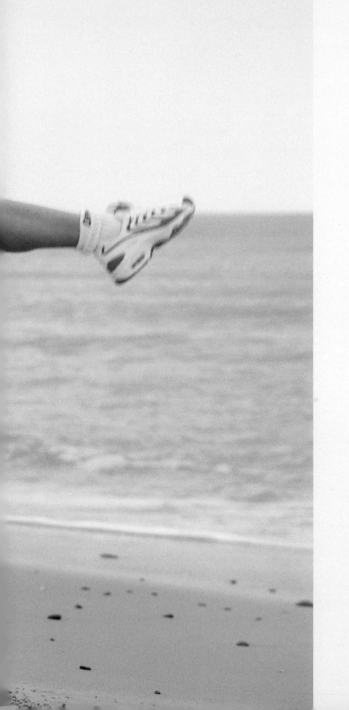

CHAPTER SEVEN

FAT-BURNING WORKOUT

It's an inescapable fact of life that women's bodies were designed to store fat because we are biologically programmed to bear children. Female reproductive organs require a certain amount of body fat to function – when body fat drops below a minimum, the menstrual cycle stops.

But that doesn't mean you can't cheat nature – just do the following workout!

The body was designed to store enough fat so that it could provide a growing baby with nutrients even in a famine. The frustrating thing for many women is that our body is following its genetic programming to the letter but we are in no danger of coming anywhere near a famine. What that means, in terms of losing fat, is that you have to do aerobic exercise – which raises your heart rate and therefore burns more calories than usual – for a long enough time (30 to 45 minutes) on a consistent basis – three to four times a week. Keep it up for at least six months, and your body will become programmed to burn fat instead of storing it. Men, on the other hand, will find that as they start to exercise, they lose fat very quickly as they do not have the same genetic programming to store it.

This workout raises the heart rate by using the body's largest muscle groups in big movements.

Different people will burn different amounts of calories by doing this workout, depending on body size and effort, but you should use up at least 300 calories in half an hour. And a safe way to lose fat is to burn 300 to 500 calories a day on most days of the week. If you do this, you will lose 14 pounds easily in ten weeks. If you do this or one of the other workouts in this book every day, and cut back on 250 calories a day (which you could do by giving up that morning cappuccino, mid-afternoon chocolate bar, or nightly half bottle of wine), you'll lose over a pound of fat a week. And that's safe, effective fat loss that you're more likely to keep off than any weight loss by a crash diet.

Another bonus is that if you work out regularly, your body becomes more efficient at burning fat even when it's at rest. That's because the trained muscle is better suited to using fat as a source of energy.

HOW DO I KNOW I AM WORKING HARD ENOUGH?

The level that we are aiming for is comfortable but challenging – during the workout you should feel hot and sweaty but still capable of having a conversation. As mentioned in chapter 1, this is an interval workout, which intersperses bouts of hard work with active recovery, allowing you to keep the activity up for a long enough time to burn a sufficient amount of calories to make a difference.

HOW LONG SHOULD I WORK OUT FOR?

Start by following the workout once through and then gradually build up to three times. You should be aiming for 30–40 minutes of cardiovascular exercise, several times a week (this also includes your warm-up and cool-down). Drink lots of water! Keep yourself hydrated during, before and after your workout.

Never stop exercising because the phone is ringing. Remember your heart rate is up and your heart busy pumping blood to all your major limbs. If you stop suddenly, that blood has nowhere to go and will end up in your lower stationary limbs leaving your head feeling dizzy and disorientated. If you have to stop, keep your feet moving and take the pace down gradually and safely.

Motivating music is a great help in getting your heart rate up – dance tracks in particular work very well. Do this to slow music, and you'll slow down, but put in a club-style mix (even if this is not your usual choice of music) and you'll work at the right rate to make a difference. You can buy mixes of club music from all the big music stores.

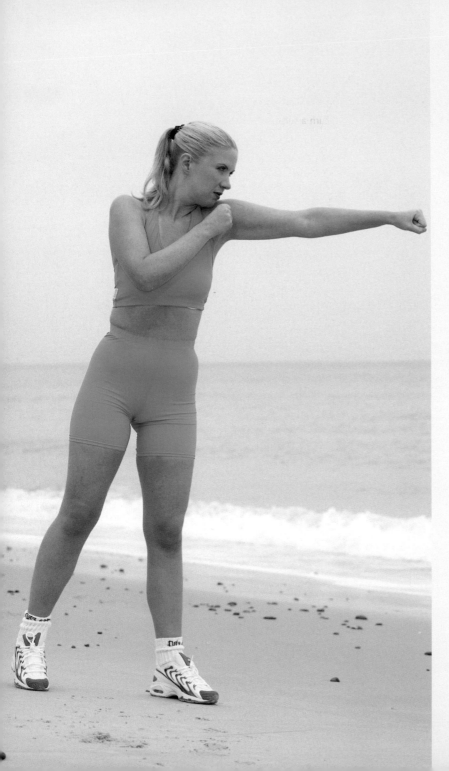

THE WORKOUT

Start with the warm up from chapter 3. When it comes to losing weight and burning calories fast, you want to get the most out of your exercise routine as possible and the more calories you burn, the better you will feel about your workout. But however eager you are to get into your fat-burning workout, do not skimp on your warm-up! Always spend at least five minutes gently warming your body up – think of your workout as a hill – spend the first part gently walking up it, warming up. The second phase, the main aerobic piece, is your walk across the top. Your cool-down is the gentle stroll back down.

- Right back kick x 20
- Front hand punch x 20
- Double side kick x 20
- Active recovery – star jumps with punches for 1–2 minutes
- Front knee raise, back leg front kick, jab and cross x 10, change legs, repeat
- Skipping – 2–5 minutes
- Active recovery
- Front hand double hook, front leg double turning kick x 10. Change legs and repeat.
- Active recovery
- Jumping knees – 1–2 minutes
- Active recovery
- Squat front kick right leg, squat front kick left leg x 20

◄

Front hand punch x 2

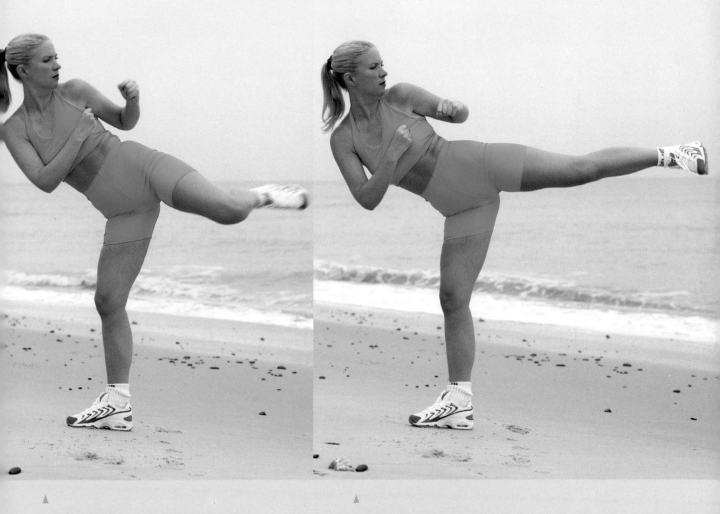

From fighting stance, right leg back kick x 20

Double side kick, right leg x 20

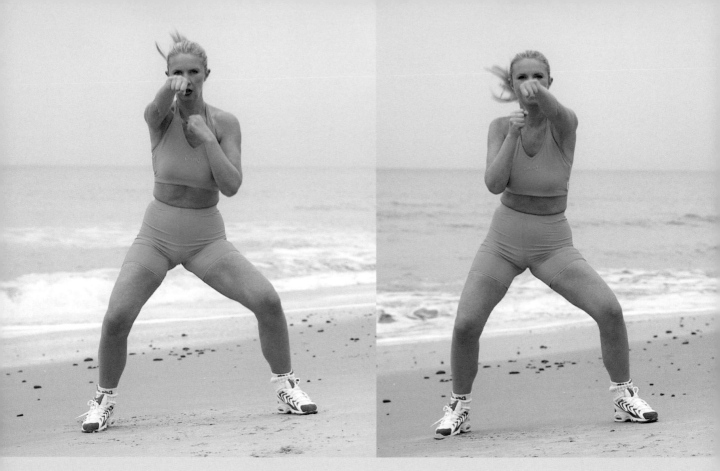

Active recovery

Star jumps with punches – jump, right hand punch, jump, left hand punch etc. for 60 seconds.

Intermediates: for up to 2 minutes.

Star jumps

It is very important to maintain good technique throughout your star jumps. Firstly, be aware that you are landing correctly – your knees should be in line with your toes and 'soft'. Do not crash-land onto the floor. Concentrate on keeping your foot-fall light. Keep your back straight and abdominal muscles firm. Your hands should be held lightly under your chin with your fists gently clenched ready to punch out alternately as you land.

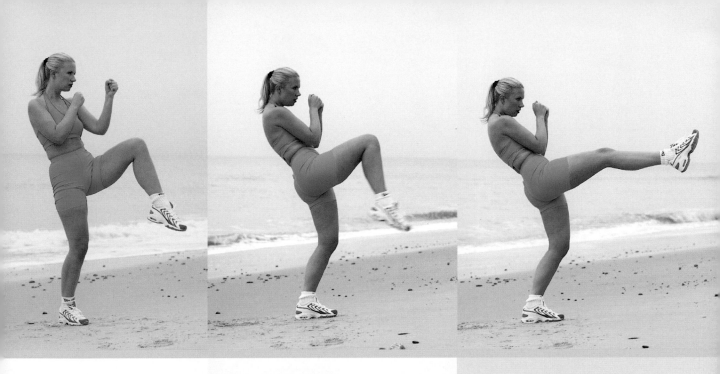

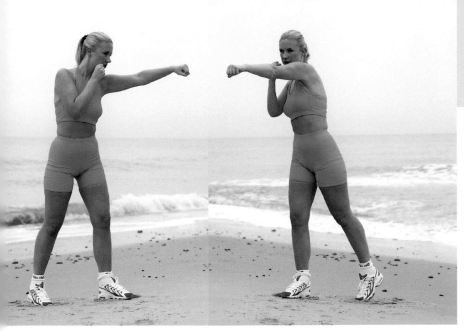

- Front knee raise, back leg front kick, jab and cross x 10. Change legs.
- Skipping for 2 minutes
- Intermediates: up to 5 minutes

Skipping

You can skip with or without a rope. However, a good skipping rope is an excellent, simple and cheap piece of aerobic equipment. Do make sure you buy a good one – and it will last you a lifetime. Skipping ropes are available from virtually all sports stockists. The main thing to check is the length – if it is either too short or too long you are going to have a problem. A lot of them are adjustable – check that it is the right length by standing on the rope with your feet shoulder-width apart. The rope should finish just under your armpits.

How to skip: sounds daft but many of us haven't skipped since school days, if then! The main problem is most people try to jump too high and put too much effort in. If you watch a martial artist or boxer skip you would be amazed at the speed and how effortless it looks. Keep your jumps as low as you can, keeping your knees and ankles soft as you land.

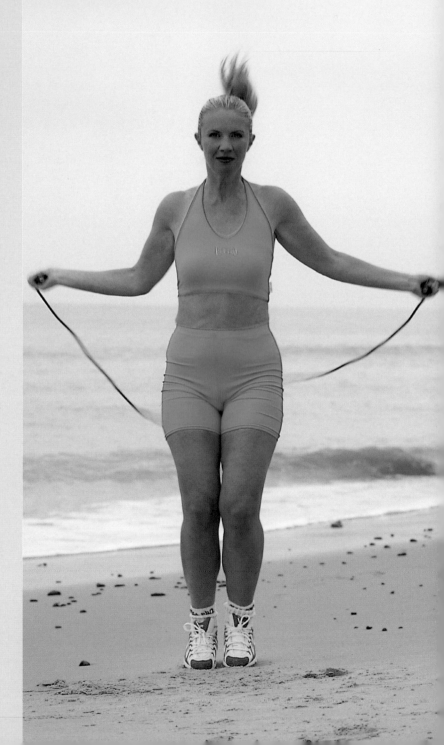

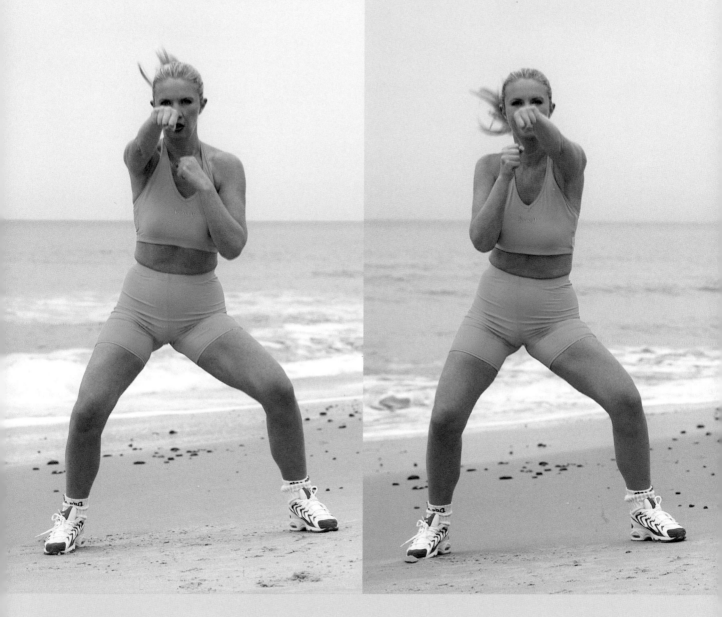

Active recovery

Star jumps with punches – jump, right hand punch, jump, left
hand punch etc. for 60 seconds.
Intermediates: for up to 2 minutes.

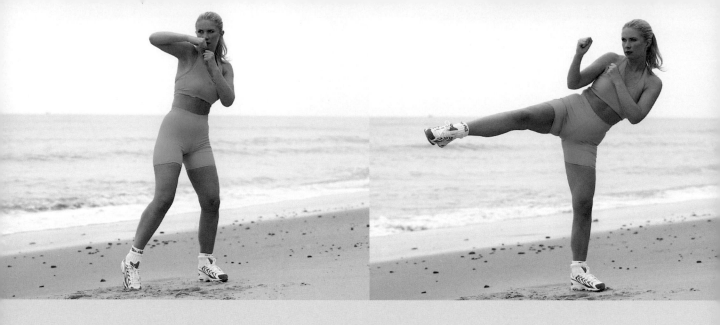

■ Front hand double hook, front leg double turning kick x 10. Change legs

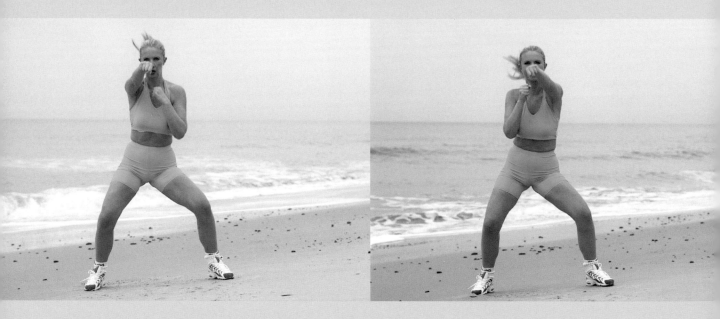

Active recovery

Star jumps with punches – jump, right hand punch,
jump, left hand punch etc. for 60 seconds.

Intermediates: for up to 2 minutes.

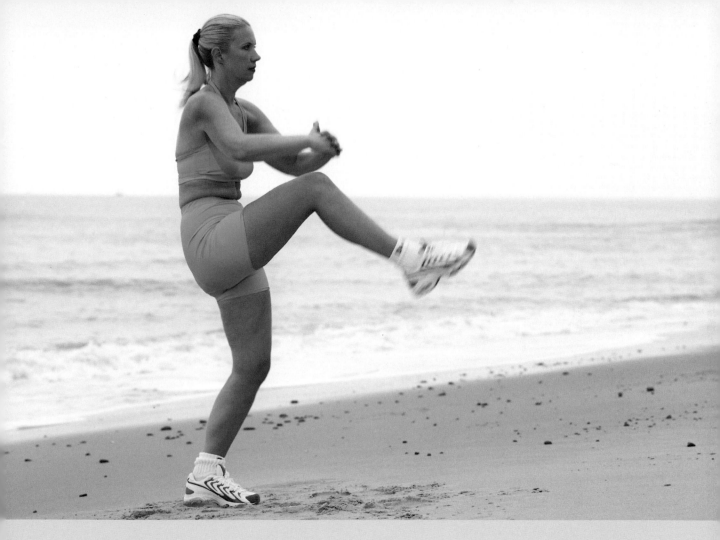

■ Jumping knees for 60 seconds (working up to 2 minutes)

Jumping knees

As with every high impact move it is important to get your landing correct. Keep your knees and ankles soft and don't crash down onto the floor. Bring your knee towards your chest keeping your back straight and your abs tight. Your knee is coming to meet your stomach, not the other way round! Reach up high with your hands before pulling them down to meet your knee.

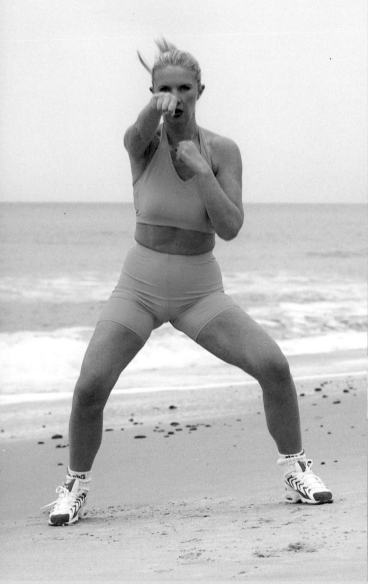
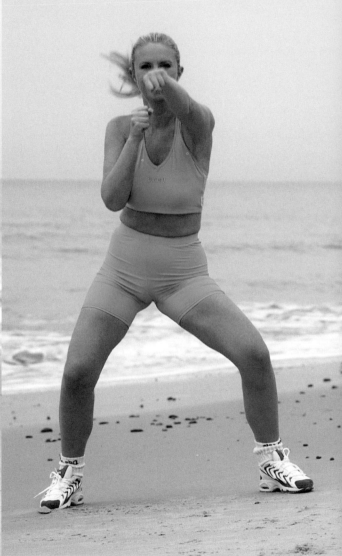

Active recovery

Star jumps with punches – jump, right hand punch,
jump, left hand punch etc. for 60 seconds.
Intermediates: for up to 2 minutes.

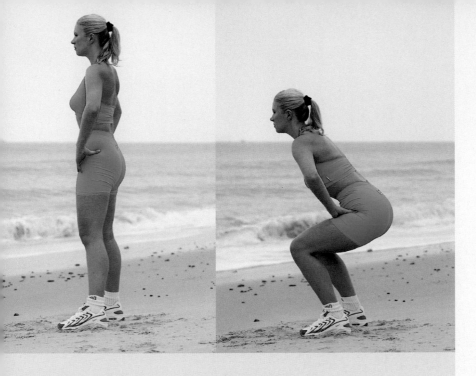

■ Squat front kick right leg – squat front kick left leg x 20

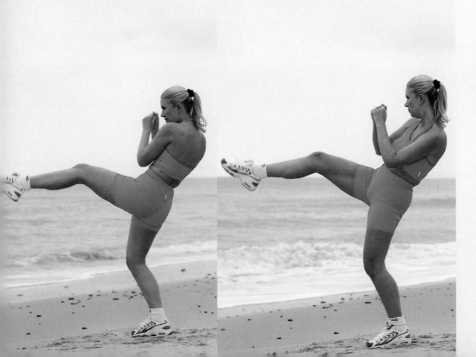

Squat kicks

Begin with your feet one-and-a-half times hip-width apart. Squat down keeping your back straight and your abs tight. Don't let your heels come off the floor and also make sure your butt doesn't travel lower than the line of your knees. As you straighten up, shift the majority of your weight onto your left supporting leg. Lift your left knee following through with a right leg front kick. Retract your kick, bringing it back into standing position and squat again. Repeat with your left leg.

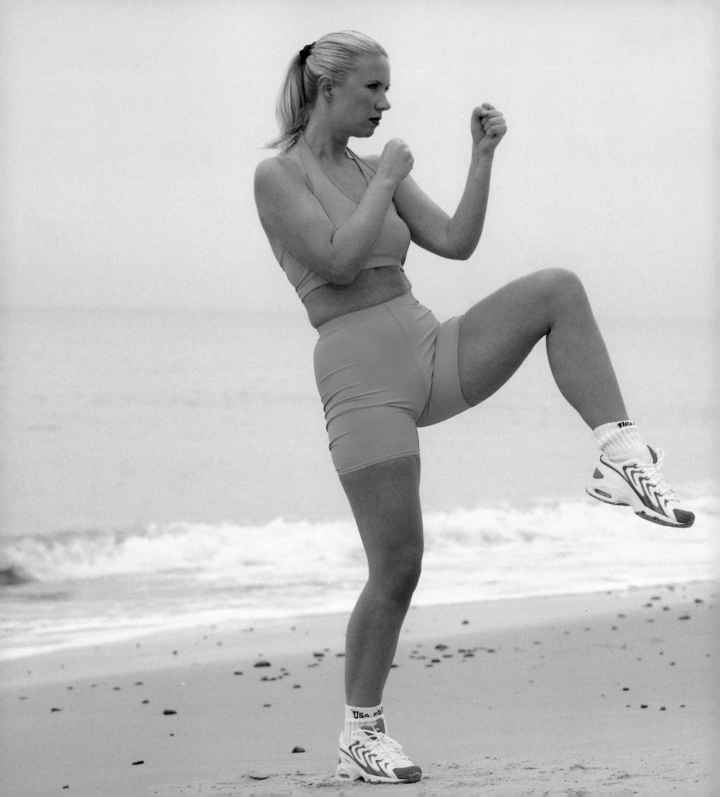

CHAPTER EIGHT

THE ABDOMINAL WORKOUT

If you pay attention to your technique – i.e. hold your abdominal muscles so that they feel engaged and strong – your abs will be conditioned by all of the workouts in this book. Your abdominals are working hard with every kick and punch, as your body is forced to engage these muscles in order to stabilize itself during these movements.

Strong abdominals are not just an essential accessory for crop tops and bikinis, they are also the core of a fit body. They support the spine, maintain good posture and can help prevent back problems. You use your abdominal muscles every time you bend down, turn your torso, or pick something up. This workout will help you work your abs in a functional way – while you are standing up and moving around – mimicking the way you use them in real life.

Gym classes tend to reserve abdominal exercises for the last five minutes of the class. While it is important to isolate these muscles for intense work by doing exercises while lying down, it is also important to be aware of them throughout every minute of the workout.

A good way to quickly improve the strength of your abs is to turn this typical scenario on its head and do your ab work at the start of your workout (immediately after your warm-up). This means that your abs will get attention before you are tired, and therefore will benefit from your best technique. Stick them on the end and you're likely to do your ab exercises with poor technique – or skip the full set altogether because you feel you have worked enough. Starting your workout with ab work also helps you to become aware of them and of how it feels when they are engaged and working, so you are more likely to continue the rest of the workout with this awareness. That means more protection for your back, more power for your kicks and punches and, in the end, abs of steel!

In the last year or two, the fitness world has reassessed the way it teaches us to train our abdominal muscles and now the focus is on the deepest abdominal muscle, the transverse abdominis. Previously, exercises had focused solely on the rectus abdominis, the muscle that runs down the front of your torso that gives the classic six-pack and enables you to curl your torso forward. But we now know that to achieve that elusive flat stomach, you also have to work the transverse abdominis, which runs horizontally in the abdominen from the lower ribs to the pubic area and acts like a corset to provide your body with that all-important core stability. A good abdominal workout also exercises the obliques, the muscles which run down the sides of the body and which rotate the spine and flex the body to the side.

HOW MANY REPS SHOULD I DO OF EACH EXERCISE?

Don't get obsessed with notching up countless repetitions – with ab work, it's quality, not quantity, that is the key. Concentrate on doing as many repetitions of each exercise with perfect technique as you can. Effective abdominal work requires concentration; it is very easy for your body to 'cheat' during these exercises. People who boast of doing 150 sit-ups in one go are very probably engaging other muscles, such as using their thighs to pull them up, or relying on momentum to power the movement, or they are pulling on the neck.

It is important to keep the neck relaxed during these exercises – your head is very heavy (it weighs nearly a stone). Keep it in line with your spine at all times, or your neck muscles will engage to support it, which will develop muscle tension and potential back problems. So aim to do as many repetitions as you can while maintaining excellent technique. That may be as little as five of each to begin with. Add to this when you feel you can do so without compromising your technique. Always end with the ab stretches.

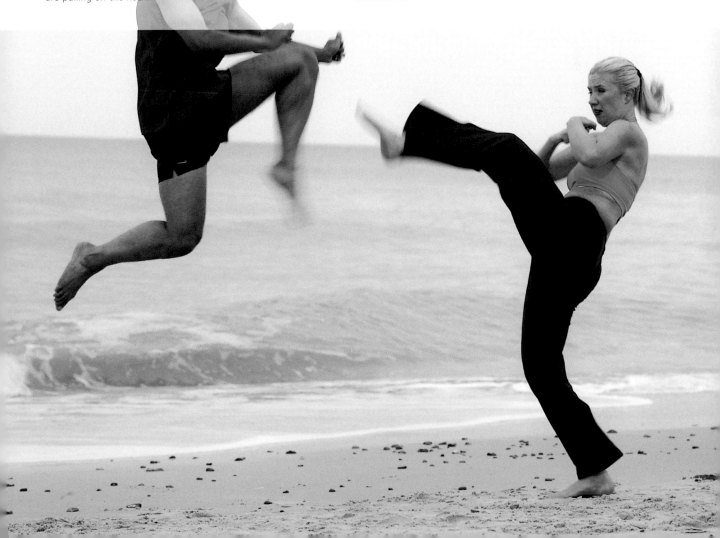

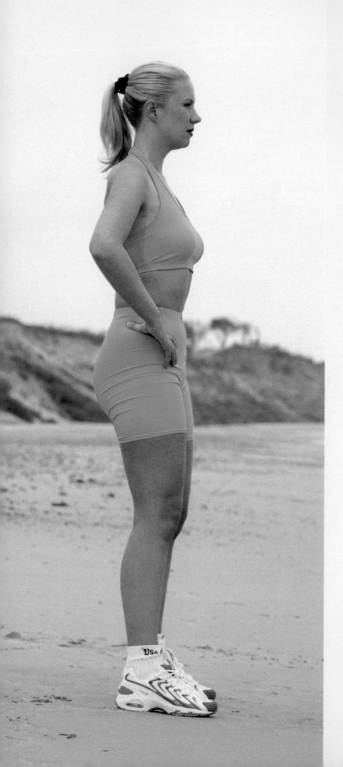

THE WORKOUT

- Abdominal curls
- Reverse curls
- Sit up and thrust
- The plank
- Oblique squeezes
- Back extensions

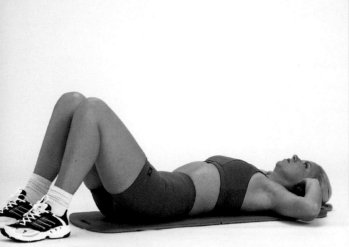
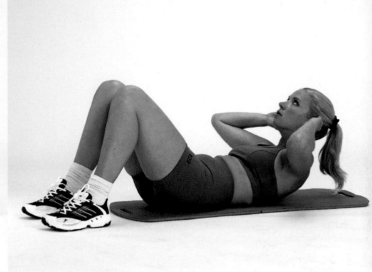

Abdominal curls

Start by lying on your back with your knees bent and feet flat on the floor. Your knees should be hip-width apart with your calf and thigh at right angles. Gently press your lower back into the floor, feeling your pelvis tip up towards you. Fix yourself into that position. Cup your head with your hands. Keeping your chin off your chest and your eyes to the ceiling, lift up while breathing out. Make sure the move is fluid and continuous. Don't just drop on the downward phase – control both up and down movements with equal care. Visualize pressing down with the muscles below your belly button whilst curling up with the ones above. Keep your lower back fixed into the floor at all times – don't arch up as you come down.

Once you have mastered the above technique and are flowing through it with ease, you can move on to a more advanced position. For an intermediate level, lift your feet off the floor, bend your knees while crossing your ankles by your butt. Again, nothing moves below the line of your belly button. Moving onto an advanced position, instead of crossing your ankles by your butt, lift your legs up until they are straight. Keep them totally still throughout the exercise.

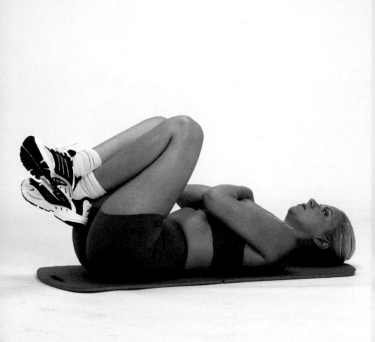
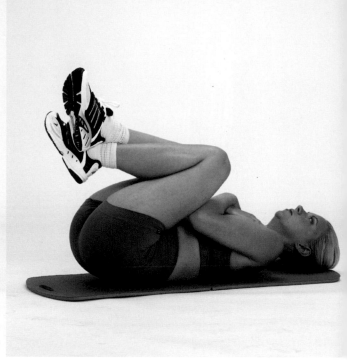

Reverse curls

Lie on your back, cross your ankles by your butt and cross your arms over your chest (this is to stop you cheating!). The idea behind this exercise is to curl your knees towards your chest, lifting your butt off the floor. It is a small move which requires control and concentration. Nothing above your belly button should move this time. Keep your upper body completely relaxed, letting the muscles below your waist line lift you up and in. Breathe out as you curl in. To make the exercise harder, lift your legs up straight above you and continue as before. Do not rock or use momentum for this exercise.

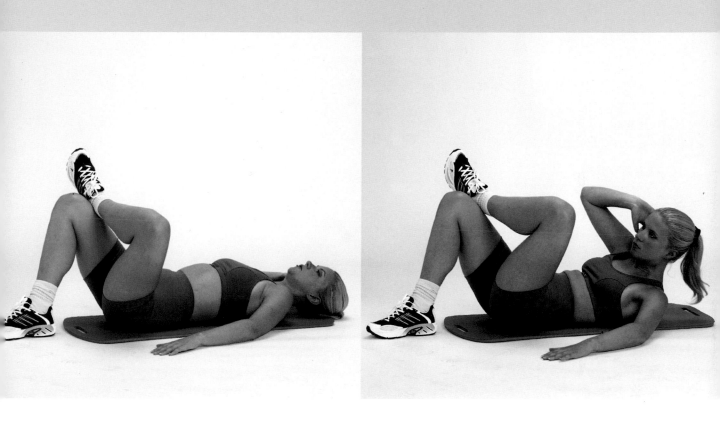

Sit-up and twists

From your original abdominal curl position, place your right ankle across your left knee keeping your hips firmly in the ground, lift and twist your left shoulder towards the right knee. Keep your chin off your chest and breathe out as you lift up. Return to the ground under control and repeat. To make this exercise harder you can take the supporting leg off the floor and 'fix' your hips and legs into place by contracting your abdominal muscles. From this position nothing should move below your hip line.

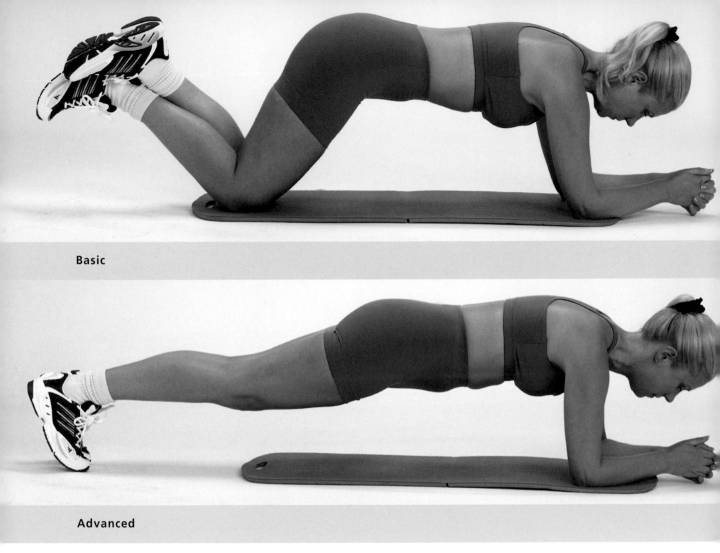

Basic

Advanced

The plank

Lie on your front with your forehead resting on your arms. Relax your body, especially your abdominals and buttocks. Inhale and as you exhale, pull your pelvic floor inwards and upwards, lifting your belly button. Hold the contraction while breathing freely for 5 seconds, building up to 30 seconds. When you feel comfortable with this, start on your forearms and knees. Contract your pelvic floor and keep your head in line with your spine. Hold for 5 to 30 seconds. Once you feel comfortable doing this, move your starting position to your arms and feet and repeat.

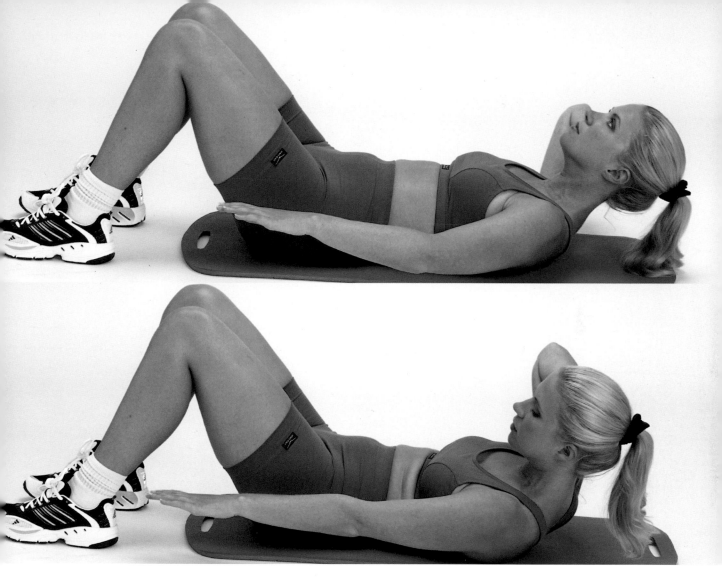

Oblique squeezes

Lie on your back with your belly button pressed to the floor. Rest your head on your right arm and extend your left arm parallel with your body. Breathe in and, pulling your abdominals in tight, reach for your left ankle with your left hand. Try to keep your shoulders parallel with the floor so that you achieve the movement by squeezing your ribs on the left side of your body to your left hip. Return to the start position and repeat before changing sides.

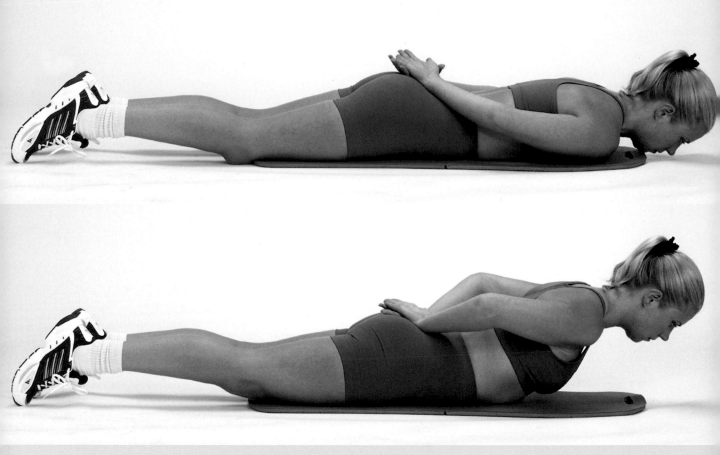

Back extensions

Lie on your front in a straight line. Take your hands to the small of your back. Relax your lower body and keep your nose towards the ground. Lift up. It is a small and controlled move using your lower back muscles. Keep the move slow and continuous trying not to tighten or clench your butt and legs. Always look down towards the ground trying to keep a straight line from the top of your head to the base of your back. It is important to maintain balance with any form of toning and strengthening programme. The lower back muscle is one that is often overlooked but also one of the most important ones to keep strong and balanced. Don't overlook it as part of your abdominal workout – they are there to help each other!

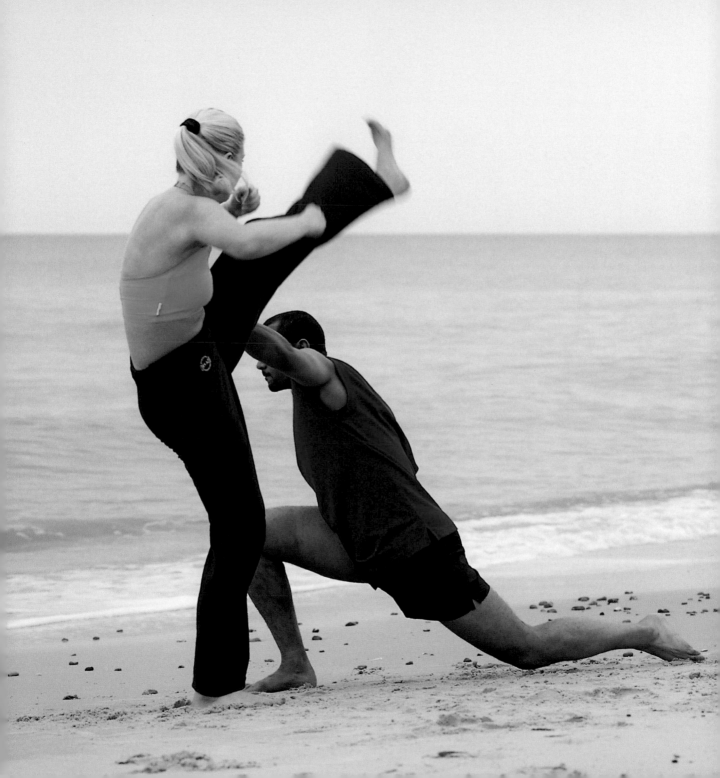

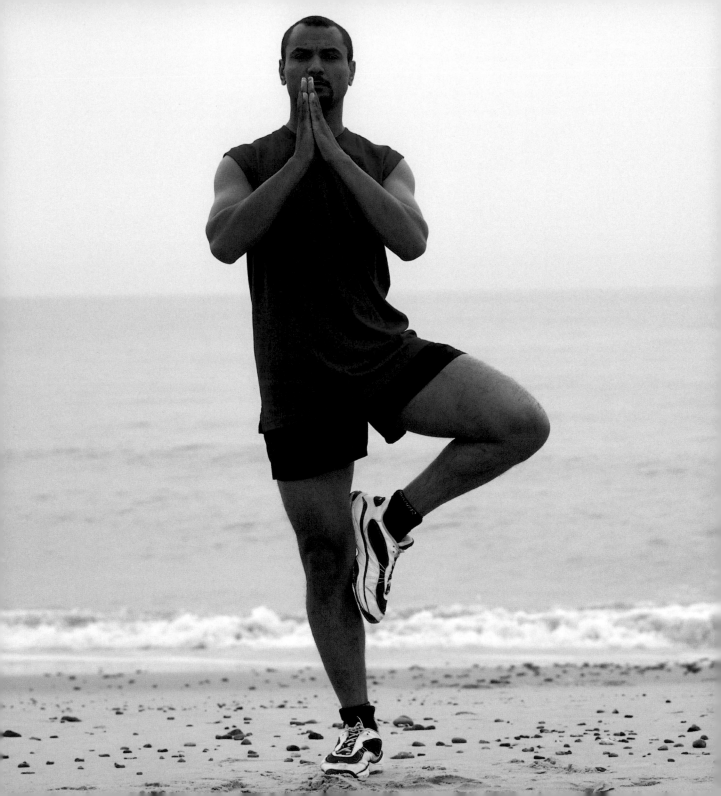

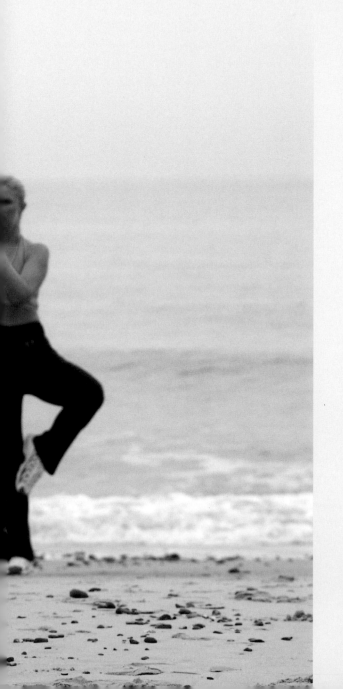

CHAPTER NINE

THE STRESS-BUSTER WORKOUT

The exercises within this workout are taken from the ancient Chinese martial arts of Tai Chi and Chi Gong. These popular and time-honoured exercises are effective for both preventive and therapeutic purposes. To get the most out of the following workout, you must try to comply with certain requirements which are unique to this system of exercise.

Firstly, keep your mind peaceful and relaxed. Focus on the exercise you are doing and not on the worries of the day. Next, combine the movements with conscious and slow breathing. Try to be aware of how every part of your body feels, this is your time to relax and shut out the world so use it well! To help you achieve this state of mind, it's helpful to do the basic relaxation exercise before you do your workout.

BASIC RELAXATION EXERCISE

Lie on your back with a pillow or other support under your head so that your head is kept straight in line with your body and therefore your spine is correctly aligned. Have your arms relaxed at your sides, your legs straight and soft and your eyes closed, your mouth shut with the upper and lower teeth touching, and the tip of your tongue placed against the roof of your mouth.

1   Breathe naturally through your nose. Regulate the breathing, keeping it steadily rhythmic in speed and depth.

2   Use a cue word to induce the relaxation response. Mentally repeat first the word 'quiet' with each inhalation, then the word 'relaxed' with each exhalation.

3   Thinking about the word 'relaxed', deliberately relax a part of your body at the same time for each breath. Start with the head, then relax in turn your arms, hands, chest, abdomen, upper back, lower back, hips and butt, legs and finally the feet. After that, scan over the whole body to see whether there are any specific areas which may still be tense. If there are, make some adjustments and allow those areas to relax.

4   Now, using the power of imagery, focus on the blood vessels, the nerves and finally the internal organs, imagining each of these to be relaxed. Try to spend at least 20 minutes on the above exercise, then move onto the following:

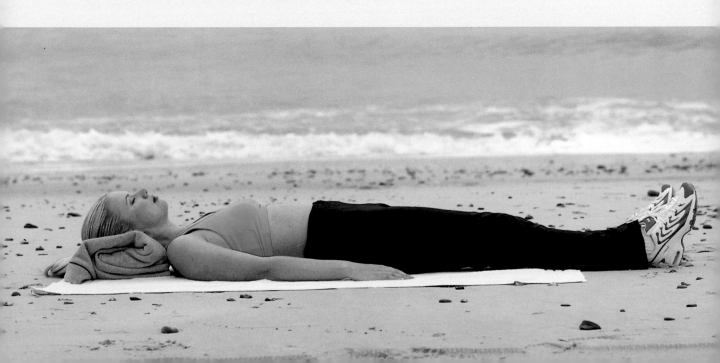

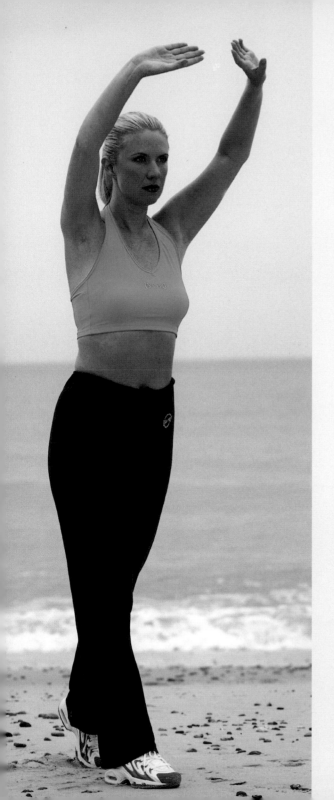

THE WORKOUT

- Arm swings
- Head circles
- Trunk twists
- Raised arm stretch
- Face rub
- Holding a ball

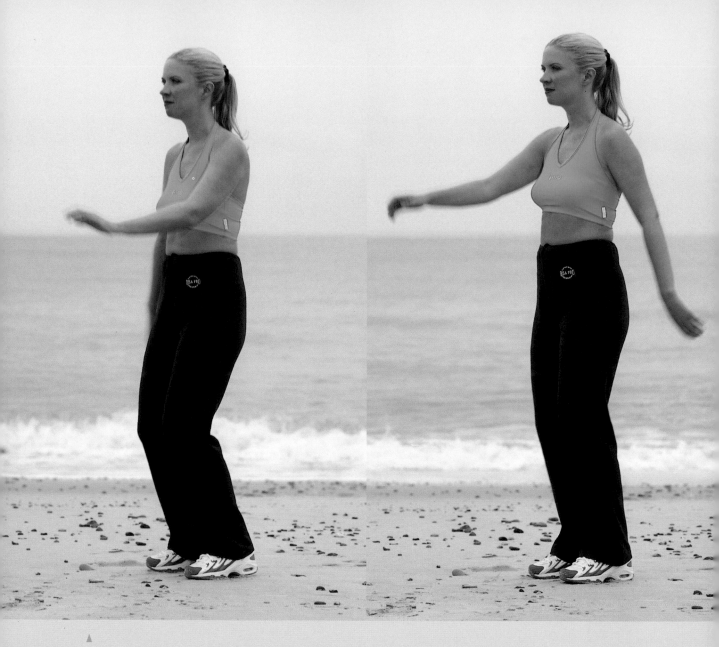

1 Stand with your feet shoulder-width apart. Swing your arms forwards and backwards, one moving forward while the other goes back. With the continuing, rhythmic swinging of the arms, sway the lower back and pelvis forwards and backwards with the same rhythm. Repeat the swinging motion for about 2 to 3 minutes.

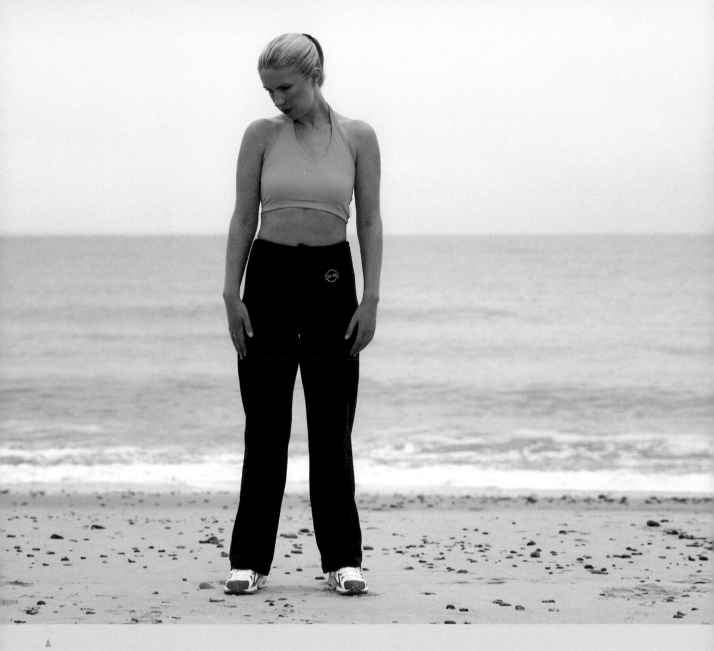

2 Still standing with your feet shoulder-width apart (though you can do this one sitting upright in a chair), bend your head forwards and then backwards. Tilt your head to the left, then to the right. Gently semi-circle the head from the left shoulder over to the right and return the same way. Do each of these moves 8 to 10 times, and then go on to the next.

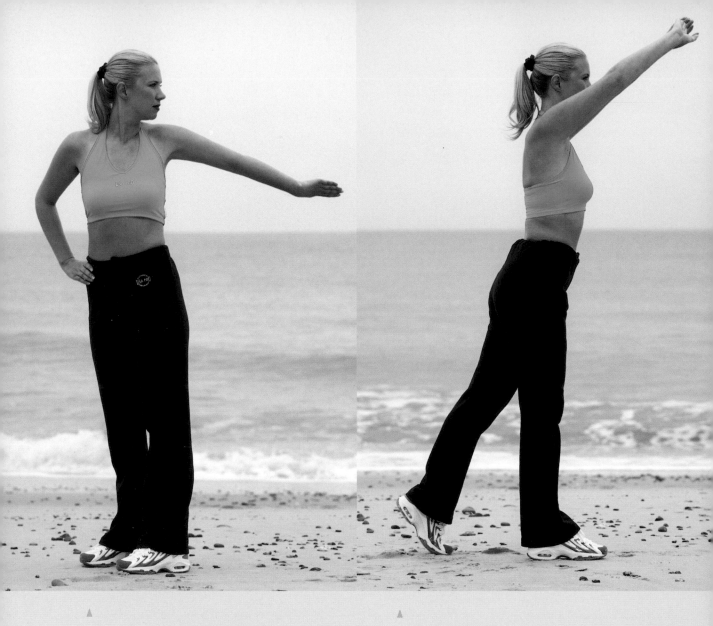

3 Still with your feet shoulder-width apart, place your hands on your hips. Twist the trunk of your body to the left and stretch the left arm horizontally backwards, elbow straight and palm upward. Return to start position and repeat in the other direction. Then return to start position. Repeat this 8 to 10 times.

4 Stand with your feet together, arms at your side. Take a step forward with your left foot and stretch both arms forward and upward. Return to starting position. Repeat with the other leg. Then again return to starting position. Repeat this 8 to 10 times.

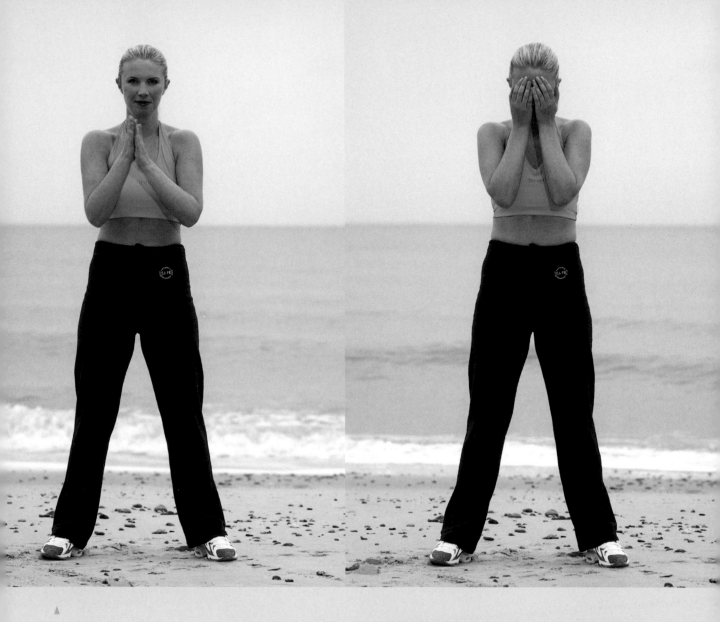

5 Rub the hands together to warm the palms. Then 'wash' the face by stroking it with your palms 20 to 30 times. Start at your chin with your fingertips and work your hands up your face through your hairline. It is said that this massage helps improve the circulation of blood to the skin, and maintains its elasticity and tone.

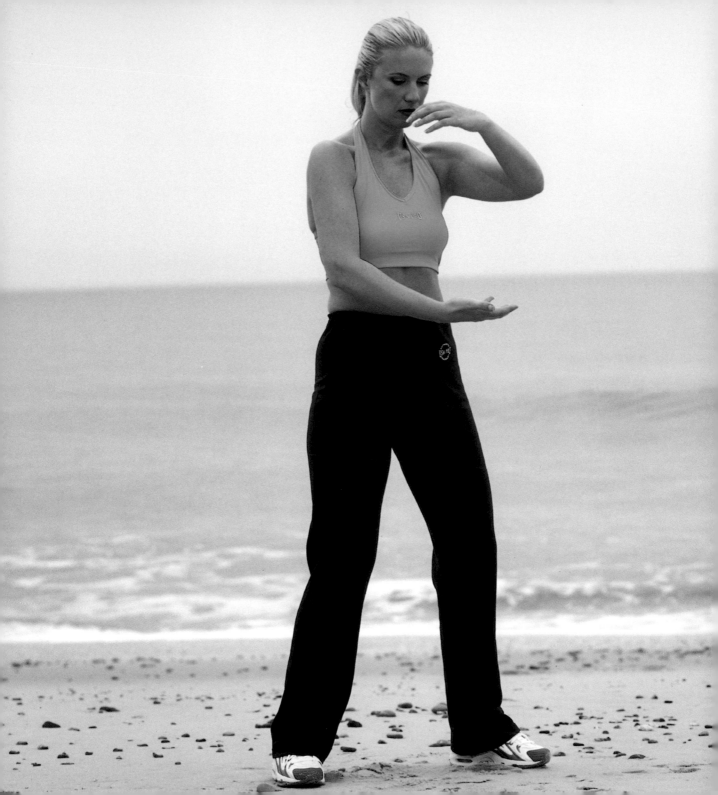

Holding a ball

Stand with your feet hip-width apart, toes pointing forwards and keep your knees soft. Raise your arms to shoulder level, bend at the elbows, as if you are holding a large ball. Move your arms round until they are holding the ball from the underneath and the top. Keep the elbows and hands relaxed and your shoulders down. Breathe deeply. Start with 30 seconds, building up to 2 minutes.

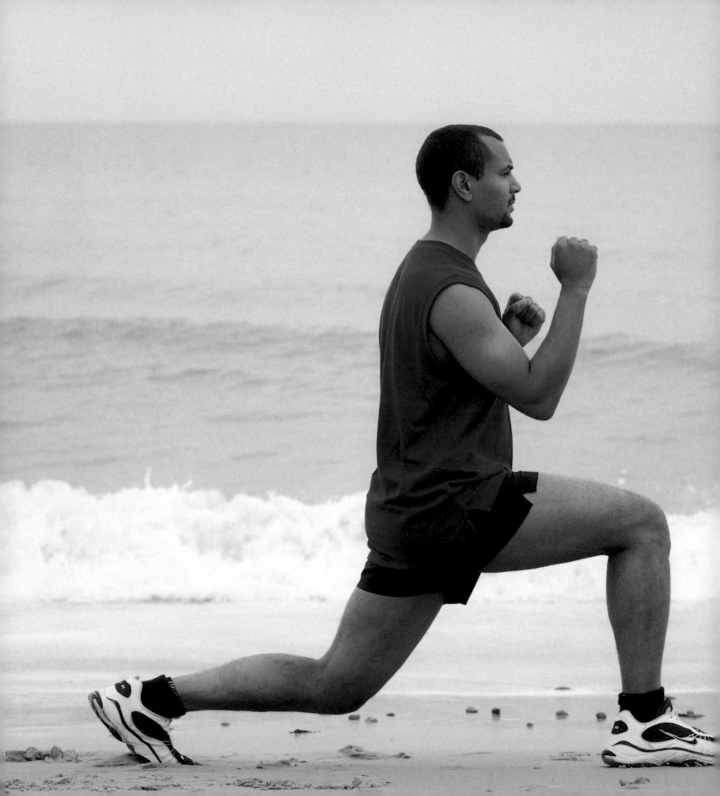

10 TIPS FOR A HEALTHY LIFESTYLE

Exercising is just one piece of a complex jigsaw; if you want to achieve optimal health and wellbeing, you have to take a holistic approach. You may think you're doing enough by simply trying to exercise regularly, and there's no doubt that it is a big achievement. But you may find, as many do, that starting to exercise regularly is a trigger for a whole chain of other changes in your life – in the very fundamentals such as the way you eat, drink and sleep.

Following is a guideline of lifestyle goals that will increase your energy levels and boost your immune system – in other words, get you glowing with health from the inside out! Don't, whatever you do, attempt to make all of these changes at once. Unless you have an iron will, you will never keep it up and will end up feeling like you've failed. Little and often is a good policy towards lots of things, including changing your life. Read and digest the following advice, but don't feel you have to put it into action until the time is right. It may take months or years, but remember, you're in this for life, so take all the time you need to make it work!

One thing that must be said, however, is that change is essential to get results. Do what you've always done, and you'll get what you've always got. If you want to get different results to those you've always got, you've got to do things differently. Here are the 10 most important changes to think about and incorporate into your life:

1 EAT WELL

Think fruit and veg first

There is a wealth of scientific evidence about the benefits of eating at least five portions of fruit and vegetables a day. They provide essential antioxidants, vitamins and minerals that your body needs to function and to fight disease (and that it can't get from a multi-vitamin supplement). Plus, it's easier than you think! All types of fruit and vegetables count: fresh, frozen, canned, dried and juiced. So, one portion could be a piece of fruit, two small fruits (such as plums or satsumas), two to three tablespoons of vegetables, a glass of juice, or a side salad. For example, if you have a glass of fruit juice with cereal and dried fruit at breakfast, fruit with lunch and as an afternoon snack, and at least two vegetables with your evening meal, you're there.

A bonus of increasing the amount of fruit and vegetables in your diet is, of course, that it leaves you less room to eat calorie-laden snacks. Here are some easy ways of sneaking extra fruit and veg into your diet:

- Buy a blender and make fruit smoothies.
- Always add salad to your sandwiches.
- Keep a fruit bowl on your desk at work for snacks.
- Keep a container of vegetable crudities (carrots, cucumber, courgettes, cauliflower) in the fridge for snacking on.
- Add a handful of frozen peas or frozen mixed vegetables to the saucepan while you are cooking pasta.
- Thinly slice peppers, broccoli, green beans or courgettes and simmer in a ready-made pasta sauce.

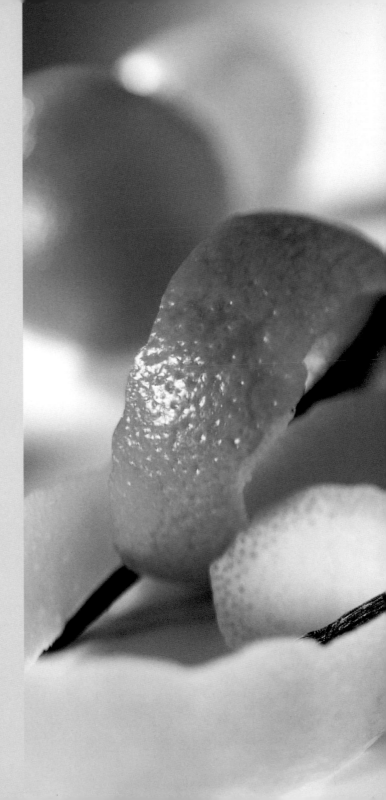

Eat breakfast

If you're one of the one in six people who doesn't eat breakfast regularly, start now! Research by nutritionists at Queen Margaret College, Edinburgh, found that a group of volunteers who were given no more dietary advice than to eat a large bowl of breakfast cereal with semi-skimmed milk every morning naturally ate less fat throughout the day and lost on average 3lbs in 12 weeks. The researchers concluded that eating breakfast can help control your weight by providing the kind of fuel for your body that releases its energy slowly and so keeps at bay mid-morning hunger pangs that can have you reaching for a chocolate bar. A low-fat/high carbohydrate breakfast (such as porridge, cereal, wholemeal toast, fruit and yoghurt) has also been shown to boost your mood.

Work out how much you're actually eating

Most of us underestimate how much we eat, partly because we overlook things like the mayonnaise in our tuna sandwich and partly because we refuse to admit that a tablespoon of cream means just that: a tablespoon, not an enormous dollop. For a more accurate calorie count, use measuring spoons and weighing scales when cooking food. A portion of pasta for instance (60g – around 200 calories) is half a mugful or about as much as you can hold in one hand. Keep a food diary for three days (including one weekend day, as most of us eat different things on Saturdays and Sundays) recording when, what and how much you ate. According to one study, people who wrote down everything they ate lost an average of half a pound a week.

Distinguish between hunger and appetite

Appetite is produced by external stimuli such as food aromas, sweets at the supermarket checkout or simply being bored, but real feelings of hunger are produced when your blood sugar levels start to fall. Unfortunately, it is easy to confuse hunger and appetite because both can cause your stomach to contract and cause you to salivate. The difference is that appetite goes away if you distract yourself with a non-food related activity such as going for a walk or cleaning your teeth. If you still feel the pangs after 20 minutes, you are hungry. If you find yourself snacking at work, keep a breath freshener spray on your desk. When you crave chocolate, give it a squirt – the minty taste takes away the desire for chocolate. Try it – it works!

Stop snacking

Give up high calorie snacks between meals and you could lose 1lb in just one week. Say you usually snack on a couple of chocolate biscuits (150 calories), a handful of peanuts (92 calories) and a Kit Kat (244 calories), that adds up to 3,400 calories a week, which converts to a whole pound of fat.

Choose wisely when eating out

We now eat out more than ever before and when you eat out, you have less control over what, and how much, you consume. The catering industry has been slow to accept that consumers want to see healthy choices on menus. However, it is possible to eat well when you eat out by following a few commonsense tips:

- Don't demolish the bread basket before your meal arrives.
- Order no more than two courses, and make sure at least one contains vegetables or fruit.
- Avoid food that is deep-fried, battered, or smothered in cheese or cream sauce.
- Be picky. Ask for your fish to be grilled or poached rather than fried, and ask for the dressing on the side when you order a salad, and for no mayonnaise with your jacket-potato filling.
- Have some alcohol-free meals every week.
- Many restaurants give huge portions to make us feel we're getting value for money. Don't feel you have to eat it all – if you hate waste, ask for a doggy bag.

Portion control is important

It doesn't matter how healthy your diet is, if you eat more calories than your body needs for energy, the excess will be stored as fat. So you snack on bags of dried fruit and nuts all day and never touch chocolate? Great for your vitamin and fibre intake, but also very high in calories. A low-fat tomato-based vegetable sauce with pasta is a balanced meal, but that doesn't mean you can eat unlimited quantities. A lot of people are still working off excess fat from the low-fat phase of the '90s, when we were told that we could eat what we wanted as long is it was low in fat. As a lot of us discovered, this is simplifying the issue.

Little and often

Most nutritionists recommend eating little and often. You shouldn't eat more than two-fists worth of food at any one sitting. When you're filling your plate with food, visualize it in your stomach. Eating smaller portions more often rather than large meals with long gaps in between is kinder on your whole digestive system.

Don't fall for fads

There has been much publicity recently over high protein, low carbohydrate diets that Hollywood celebs swear by for fast weight loss. The reason this diet does result in weight loss is simply because it's a low calorie diet (you're mainly eating fish, chicken, fruits and vegetables).

In fact, most of us eat enough protein and nutritionists advise against increasing it at the expense of carbohydrate (eating too much protein over a long period of time can damage our digestive process and has been linked with bowel cancer). Carbohydrate is your body's fuel source and without it you'll find it hard to exercise regularly. Of course, if you eat too much carbohydrate, you'll store it as fat – but that applies to all foods you eat, including protein!

Learn more

For more information on healthy eating read *Body Foods for Life* by Jane Clarke.

2 DRINK LOTS OF WATER

No supermodel is ever without her 2-litre bottle of mineral water, and when interviewed, they will invariably cite drinking lots of water as their best health and beauty tip. Whatever you may think about the health advice of your average walking clothes-horse, they did cotton on to the benefits of drinking lots of water long before the rest of us.

Water keeps your digestive system working efficiently, helping you to metabolize fat and get rid of toxins. It also boosts your energy levels and, according to one study, helps your concentration (sip a glass of water throughout your next meeting and see if it improves your performance!). However, the body's thirst response is relatively slow – so by the time you feel 'thirsty', you are already dehydrated. The key is to avoid ever feeling thirsty by keeping your hydration levels topped up.

Ideally, you should aim to drink 2 to 3 litres of plain water (fizzy drinks, fruit juices and tea and coffee don't count) a day, and more if you are very active. If you are not used to doing this, you will find that you are never out of the bathroom at first, but your body will soon settle down into a normal pattern (and incidentally, a good indicator of your hydration levels is the colour of your urine: the clearer it is, the better). Women often find that they store more water at first, so don't give up if you feel bloated for the first couple of weeks. Drinking more water will ultimately help you eliminate water retention.

Get into the habit of having a glass of water as soon as you get up in the morning, to replace the fluid lost throughout the night (we lose water every time we breathe out through evaporation). Some people swear by drinking warm (i.e. boiled and slightly cooled) water with a slice of lemon first thing for getting the metabolism working. Keep a 2-litre bottle of water with you on your desk (or with you as you go about your day) and make sure you finish it. Always ask for a bottle of mineral water in restaurants and drink it alongside your wine (or instead of the wine!).

A word about fizzy (carbonated) drinks: we are consuming more and more and the choice is ever-expanding, but according to a recent study, consuming more than five cans a day can put the health of your bones at risk. These drinks leech the calcium from bones, especially in women, and experts are predicting that a whole generation of girls are growing up at risk of osteoporosis, brittle bone disease, because they drink too many fizzy drinks.

3 THROW AWAY THE SCALES

Would you let a plastic and metal object that costs around £10 ($15) to buy and probably £1 to make dictate whether you will feel happy or not on any given day? Sounds ridiculous, yet thousands of us have precisely this relationship with our bathroom scales. We choose a figure that we decide is our ideal weight and whether the needle falls to the left or right of it when we step on the scales in the morning will dictate our mood for the rest of the day.

It's time we rebelled against the tyranny of weighing scales. It's not just women who are suffering – a growing number of men step on the scales every day and bemoan the fact that despite their best efforts they're not bulking up (in the US, there's even a name for it: 'bigorexia'.) The best thing you can do for your self-esteem and to build body confidence, is to throw them out today. They serve absolutely no purpose at all. If a woman is tall she can weigh 11 stone (154lbs) and she'll look slim and have a healthy BMI (body mass index or weight to height ratio).

It is now thought that waist measurement is the most accurate indicator of health. A waist measurement of over 32in on an average-sized woman is likely to be a health risk. If it's over 35in, the risk is substantially increased.

Many women are distressed to find that when they start exercising, they start to weigh more. This is another reason why weighing scales are useless. As you get fitter, you will lose body fat, and gain lean muscle tissue. But muscle weighs more than fat, so your weight on the scales will go up, even though your body is becoming slimmer. Size is a much better indicator of results: go by the way your clothes are fitting. If they're getting looser, and you're dropping a dress size, then you're getting results – whatever it says on the scales. For a more accurate record, measure your thighs, hips, waist and chest and record the figures in your training diary. Then re-measure after every four weeks and record your progress.

4 GET ENOUGH SLEEP

'Sleep debt' is the health industry's newest buzzword, and it's been blamed for a whole host of negative effects from weight gain to ageing. The theory is that most of us don't get enough sleep on a regular basis, and accumulate a sleep debt over time which is detrimental to health. But whether this is indeed the case, it is true that sleep is essential for our survival.

While we're asleep, our brains go through a series of 90-minute cycles, and each cycle takes us through five stages of sleep. Stage one is a very light, drowsy sleep; stage two is a moderately light sleep; stages three and four are the deepest, most physically restful form of sleep, known as deep or slow-wave sleep; the concluding stage is rapid eye movement (REM) or dream sleep. In this final stage, our body is paralysed (to stop us acting out our dreams) but our eyes move rapidly under closed lids and our brain waves are active. It is generally thought that bodily repair takes place in deep sleep and brain repair in REM sleep. Regeneration cannot happen while we're awake because the energy needed for it is siphoned off elsewhere. So if you don't get enough deep and REM sleep, you'll feel physically and mentally exhausted.

So how much sleep is ideal? Ninety-five per cent of people sleep between six to ten hours a night, and the average is eight hours a night. Most people do not thrive on less than six hours sleep a night. But good-quality sleep is becoming elusive for many of us (referrals to the Sleep Disorders Centre in St Thomas's Hospital, London, have more than trebled in the past seven years.) Here are their basic tips for better sleep:

- Don't go to bed straight after a heavy meal (wait about two hours) or on an empty stomach (have a light snack, such as a milky drink or a small bowl of cereal). A stimulant such as caffeine can cause leg movements and twitching which, even if you don't wake up, may impair the quality of your sleep.
- Go to bed at a regular time, making sure your bedroom's not too hot or too cold, that there's enough ventilation.
- Don't work out too late at night.
- Rid your mind of worries. If you can't switch off, try writing down what's bothering you then leave it in a different room from the one you're sleeping in.
- Try a few drops of lavender essential oil on your pillow – it's an ancient remedy for insomnia.
- Regular exercise promotes sleep – and not only because a tired body wants to rest. Exercise increases the temperature of the brain, making it sleepy.

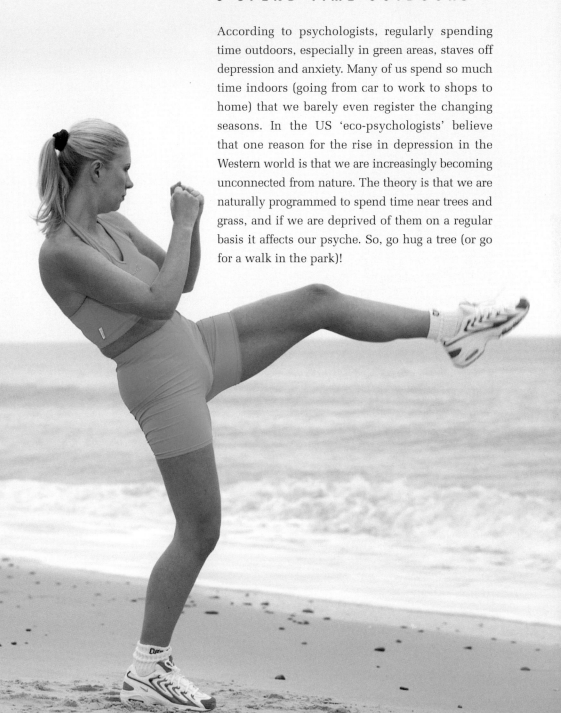

5 SPEND TIME OUTDOORS

According to psychologists, regularly spending time outdoors, especially in green areas, staves off depression and anxiety. Many of us spend so much time indoors (going from car to work to shops to home) that we barely even register the changing seasons. In the US 'eco-psychologists' believe that one reason for the rise in depression in the Western world is that we are increasingly becoming unconnected from nature. The theory is that we are naturally programmed to spend time near trees and grass, and if we are deprived of them on a regular basis it affects our psyche. So, go hug a tree (or go for a walk in the park)!

Women take one-third less exercise today than they did a generation ago, thanks to the widespread increase in labour-saving devices. According to research by Gail Goldberg, a scientist at the Dunn Clinical Nutrition Centre in Cambridge, UK, this is the prime cause of obesity. She estimates '50s shoppers spent ten hours and 2,400 calories a week walking from shop to shop, while today's shopper burns a mere 276 calories a week driving to the supermarket and wheeling around a trolley. Goldberg even believes using a cordless phone cuts down walking in the home by ten miles a year, and making a bed with a duvet instead of blankets uses up around 300 fewer calories a week. To increase your activity levels, try this trick. Throw away your remote control and get out of your chair to change channels. For a 10st 7lb person, the 12ft round trip between the sofa and TV, five times daily, should burn an extra 130 calories a day (or a KitKat!).

Human beings were designed to be active, and rather than making us feel tired, the more activity in your life, the more energy you will have. Oxygen is our life source, and exercise helps us get more of it in our bodies. Increased blood flow transports more oxygen around the body, stimulates toxin drainage through the lymphatic system and helps eliminate waste products in the muscles. Endorphins, the brain's feel-good chemicals are released into the bloodstream and after a while they reach the brain. The fitter you are, the more energy you will have. This is because your body becomes more efficient at pumping blood, and you utilize your full lung capacity. More blood flow to the brain improves alertness and memory.

Your weekly exercise sessions are vital, but they should be the icing on the cake of an active life, rather than the only activity in an otherwise sedentary existence. That means leaving the car at home and walking as much as possible, and walking up stairs instead of taking the lift or escalator.

7 FIND A WAY OF RELAXING

Long-term psychological stress impairs the efficiency of our immune system and can make us vulnerable to illness. Modern life requires a certain tolerance to stress on a daily basis – whether it's caused by your journey to work, the queue at the supermarket or that late deadline – it is often something we cannot control. But we can control our response to the situation. You can allow yourself to become tense, anxious or irritated by a situation or you can accept that giving in to those feelings won't change the situation, but will leave you feeling bad. Taking deep breaths is an amazingly simple way of calming yourself down.

Try to find a way of relaxing every day. That doesn't mean slumping in front of the TV, which is not truly relaxing, to resorting to alcohol and smoking. Instead, take a 20-minute bath with some lavender essential oil, listen to your favourite music, weed the garden, sit outside and look at the trees and read *Don't Sweat the Small Stuff (and it's all Small Stuff)* by Richard Carlson.

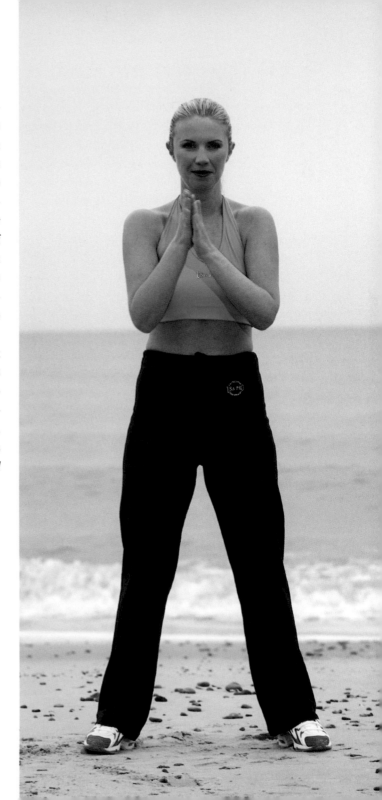

8 LAUGH EVERY DAY

Smiles and laughter trigger the release into your body of endorphins, feel-good chemicals which help you relax and feel more optimistic about life. Ben Renshaw of the Happiness Project recommends this exercise:

Sit or stand in front of a large mirror and try smiling at yourself. At first, it may be difficult to do and feel a bit false but persevere and keep on smiling. Once you are able to force a smile, take a few long, deep breaths in and out and relax as you continue smiling. It will soon start to seem more natural and you'll immediately notice how much more relaxed and optmistic you feel.

9 GIVE UP SMOKING

If you're a smoker, you're probably expecting the usual doom and gloom report here that you have read a million times before '... heart disease, blah blah, lung cancer, blah blah blah.' At which your eyes will glaze over and the part of your pysche labelled 'denial' that has convinced you that these statistics don't apply to you will kick in. So instead, here's the good news: Just 24 hours after quitting smoking, carbon monoxide is eliminated from the body and the lungs begin to clear out debris. After 72 hours, breathing becomes easier and energy levels increase, and smokers who quit before the age of 35 enjoy a similar life expectancy to people who have never smoked.

A word here about 'light' cigarettes such as Silk Cut Ultra and Marlboro Lights. You may think you are reducing the health risks by opting for cigarettes labelled 'low-tar'. Tobacco companies are certainly profiting from this generally held impression. But although the tar and nicotine in these cigarettes is made less concentrated by the presence of more filters, the increase of sales of these products has coincided with the appearance of a previously very rare form of cancer called adeno carcinoma, a form of lung cancer that strikes deep in the lungs. Cancer specialists think this is because smokers take deeper inhalations and more puffs per cigarette to get the required nicotine hit. Incidentally, they also believe that the tobacco industry has been aware of this for some time.

But giving up smoking isn't easy (is that possibly the understatement of the year?) so give yourself as much help as you need. Using a nicotine replacement therapy (NRT) such as a patch, gum or inhaler can greatly increase your chances.

10 DRINK SENSIBLY

The dangers of excessive drinking have been just as well documented, especially 'binge drinking' – being 'good' all week, then drinking all of your week's alcohol units on a Friday or Saturday night. But if this doesn't motivate you to cut down, maybe this will: alcohol is so high in calories it should be called 'liquid cake'. If you gave up alcohol for two weeks and you normally drink 14 units a week, going on the wagon will have saved you 2,600 calories – that's nearly one whole pound of fat.

A bottle of wine has around 1000 calories and a can of lager 200 calories – take a look at the empties by your kitchen bin waiting to be recycled and work out how many calories you've consumed and stored in your body. If you have several glasses of wine followed by a meal, your body will use the calories from the wine for energy, as alcohol calories are very easily converted and offer no nutritional value, which means that the calories you take in afterwards when you eat (and studies show that we tend to eat more while drinking) will be stored as fat. Don't let this be a reason to think, OK, when I'm on a bender I won't eat then! Alcohol supplies energy without any nutrients, and in fact, the processing of alcohol will cost your body nutrients. So a liquid diet supplies nothing more to your body than calories. Get into the habit of having regular alcohol-free evenings and, if you do want to lose a few pounds, there's no more effective way of doing it than giving up drinking for a while.

Weight issues aside, alcohol is a depressant so although getting drunk may be fun at the time, it will leave you feeling low the next day. You may have read the reports last year that drinking one glass of wine a day can reduce your risk of heart disease. This is true, but unfortunately, unless you are a post-menopausal woman, your risk of heart disease is not very high anyway!

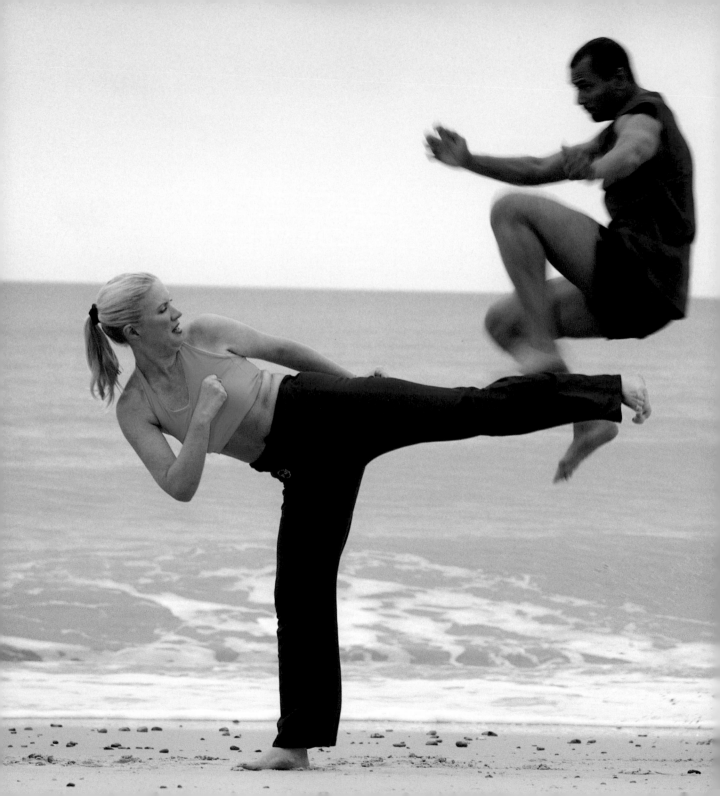

MOVING ON

We hope that *Kick Your Way to Fitness* has given you a taste of exercising martial arts-style. If it has inspired you to learn more about pure martial arts, there are plenty to choose from – so you'll be able to find a style that suits you.

To learn more about Fusion Fitness, the style I have developed and which you've seen in this book, you can contact a Fusion Fitness personal trainer:

Fusion Fitness
99 Middle Lane
London
N8 8NX

Tel: 020 8374 6087
www.fusionfit.com

MARTIAL ARTS

With such a range of martial arts to choose from, it's worth looking around at what's available in your area before you settle on a style. You'll find that dojos (martial arts gyms) will welcome you in to watch a few classes and see what goes on there. Try to get a feel for the atmosphere, if it seems friendly and welcoming to beginners. Ask a few questions, such as:

What are the instructors' qualifications?
What are the levels of contact in sparring (most contact is reserved for competitions and the level of contact is predetermined as one of three levels: light, medium or full)?
Is there a beginners' class?
Does the club have personal injury insurance?

There are numbers for specific styles of martial arts under the following headings, but a good starting point is often an umbrella organization:

UK
The Martial Arts Foundation

PO Box 18253
London EC1N 8FY

Tel: 020 7713 5779
Fax: 020 7713 5889
E-mail: contact@martialartsfoundation.org; or visit the website: www.martialartsfoundation.org.

Amateur Martial Association (AMA)

120 Cromer Street
London WC1H 8BS
Tel: 020 7837 4406

British Council of Chinese Martial Arts

c/o 110 Frensham Drive
Stockingford
Nuneaton
Warwickshire CV10 9Ql
Tel: 01203 394642

AUSTRALIA
Martial Arts World

265 Victoria Road
Gladesville
Syndey
Australia

Or, PO Box 334
Gladesville
Sydney 2111
Australia
Tel: 61 (02) 8163 7777

Martial Arts World, www.ozemail.com.au/~maworld/ has links to 318 organizations throughout Australia, as well as mail order supplies of uniforms, accessories, equipment and books.

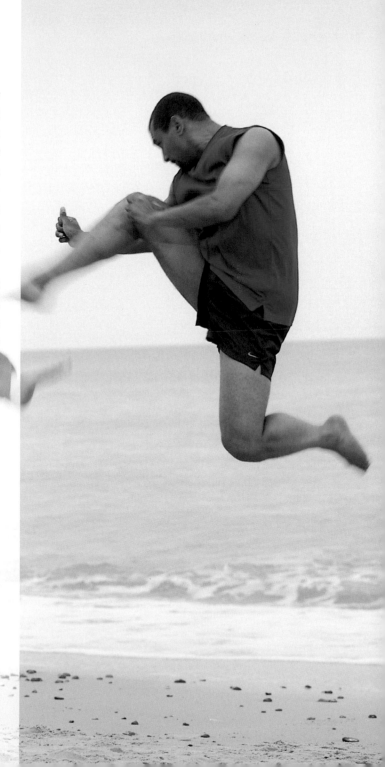

USA

The World Martial Arts League was founded by American soldiers, stationed in Japan, Okinawa and Korea. These servicemen used their time to learn Karate and when they returned brought their Martial Arts to the U.S.A. and Europe. Between 1927 and 1960, (in the beginning of this organization), some Japanese grandmasters accepted the invitations of their students and travelled to the U.S.A. to hold seminars and give demonstrations. Contact: www.angelfire.com/ks/wmal

Or visit the Martial Arts Network Online at www.tman.com – a well-organised and professional site that has comprehensive links to organizations offering all styles of martial arts throughout the world, as well as a mail order facility for books, clothing and equipment. Or contact by mail at:

1000 Universal Studios Plaza
Building 22
Orlando
Florida 32819
Tel: 07 370 4460

AIKIDO

Originating from Ju-jitsu and resembling Tai Chi in its application, Aikido uses quick and calculated movements in defensive strategies. Offensive kicks and punches are rarely applied. Instead the Aikido artist moves in the direction of the opponent with flowing circular actions. Using his own energy and momentum the opponent is thrown and blocked with graceful effortlessness.

The two goals of Aikido are to overcome the opponent and to throw the opponent. To this end, hundreds of combinations are learned in prepared sequences. Aikido also includes basic sword and staff techniques, although the significance of weapons in the art has diminished somewhat.

UK
British Aikido Board

6 Halkingcroft
Langley
Slough SL3 7AT
Tel: 01753 577878

British Aikido Federation

BAF Head Office
Yew Tree Cottage
Toot Baldon
Oxford OX44 9NE
Tel: 01865 343500
Website: www.ai-ki-do.org.uk

USA
Aikido Association of America

1016 W. Belmont Ave
Chicago, Il
60657 USA
Tel: 773 525 3141
E-mail: AikidoAmer@aol.com

Aikido Association International

945 N. Rand Road
Arlington Heights, Il
60004 USA
Tel: 847 797 1437

AUSTRALIA

The National Aikido Association of Australia has contact details of dojos throughout the country.

GPO Box 2783 EE
Melbourne
Australia 3001
Website: www.labyrinth.au/~aikido

CAPOEIRA

A Brazilian martial art developed by the descendants of African slaves, Capoeira is quite unique. It is the most acrobatic and contortionist of fighting forms and involves music. Opponents take turns delivering mostly kicks, while using their hands for support on the floor. It is a style that incorporates dance, gymnastics and fighting in one.

UK

The London School of Capoeira
45 Lorne Road
London N4 3RU
Tel: 020 7281 2020

USA AND WORDWIDE

Contact www.capoeiranyc.com for clubs throughout the States and worldwide.

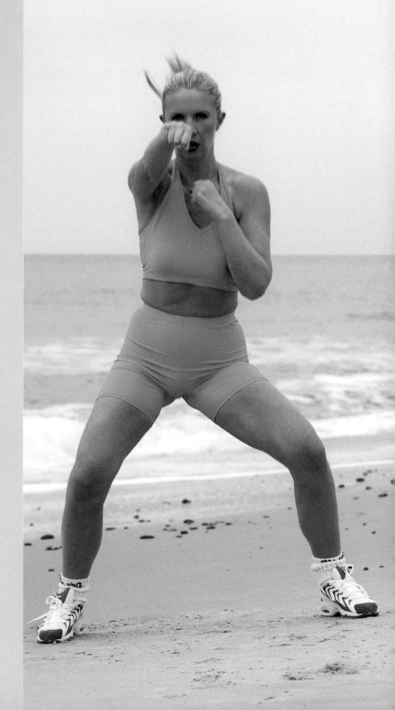

JUDO

This extremely popular sport is a modern development in martial arts. Its roots lie in Ju-jitsu, almost exclusively adopting the essential elements of subduing opponents with throws and holds. Stance and balance are important, as well as flexibility and agility.

Again the emphasis is on defensive rather than aggressive fighting strategies that use the opponent's momentum and energy against him. Additionally, knowledge of the body's vital points, for joint twists and locks are fundamental for a successful Judo artist. Much Judo action happens at ground level; combatants using their own force and weight against each other.

UK
British Judo Association

7A Rutland Street
Leicester LE1 1RB
Tel: 0116 255 9669

USA
United States Judo

15119 Mermaid Drive
Suite 101
Houston
Texas 77079-4326
Tel: 713 558 9997
Website: www.usjudo.org

Or try the World Judo Organization webiste:
www.worldjudo.org/usaclubs

AUSTRALIA
Judo Federation of Australia

PO Box 919
Glebe
NSW 2037
Tel: 61 29566 2063
Website: www.ausport.gove.au/judo

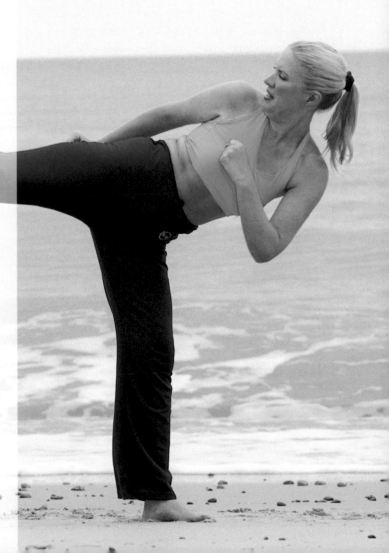

JU-JITSU

This style, sometimes known as the father of Japanese martial arts, evolved over centuries to also influence Aikido and Judo. Ju-jitsu was originally developed by Samurai warriors to compliment their skills with weapons.

The composition of moves is varied, including kicking, striking, kneeing, choking, joint locking and immobilisation. The relative strength of the opponents is made irrelevant by knowledge of the body's vital points. Maximum results are produced from what seems like minimal physical effort, when the opponents own momentum and force is used against him.

UK

The British Ju-Jitsu Association Governing Body
5 Avenue Parade
Accrington
Lancs BB5 6PN
Tel: 0114 266 6733

USA

Ju-Jitsu Federation of the US
United St
3816 Bellingham Drive
Remo NV 89511
USA
Website: www.usjujuitsu.net

AUSTRALIA

Australian And International Ju-Jitsu and Karate
PO Box 134
Ascot Vale
Victoria
Australia 3032
Tel: 61-30 9375 7444
Website: www.mira.net

KARATE

This is a relatively new style developed on the island of Okinawa, Japan. Unlike many of the other Japanese martial arts, this fighting technique was not developed and used by Samurai warriors but by humble farmers and fishermen who needed to defend themselves against invasion and attack.

The punches and strikes are characterised by spearlike thrusts of the hands, the fingers bent in various fashions to give different types of blows. Kicking is also used, as well as defensive blocks and what have become famous breaking techniques.

The objective of karate is efficiency of movement, attacks come in straight lines and actions are kept short, sharp and direct. Due to its humble origins and 'hard' nature, Karate is perhaps the least philosophically influenced of the martial arts.

UK
English Karate Governing Body

58 Bloomfield Drive
Bath
Avon BA2 2BG
Tel: 01225 834008

T'ien ti tua Ch'uan-Shu:

A respected academy established in 1975 by Mike Symonds.
Tel: 01603 665159
Website: www.kungfu.fg.co.uk

USA
United States Karate Federation

1300 Kenmore Drive Blvd
Akron
Ohio 44310
Tel: 330 753 3114
Website: www.usakarate.org

AUSTRALIA
Australian Academy of Martial Arts

A karate school operating out of South East Queensland, with links to the rest of the country.
Website: www.kodmon.com.au/aama/

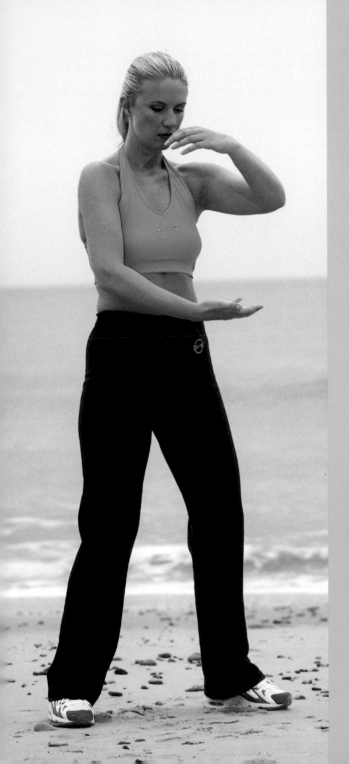

KENDO

Kendo is a highly evolved form of Japanese sword fighting practised for centuries by the Samurai and Bushi warriors. The art of Kendo is perhaps the most ritualized of all martial arts. The putting-on and taking-off of the protective armour are highly choreographed activities. This ritual prepares and relaxes the fighter for a loud and furious exchange of lightning strikes. Flexible bamboo swords have evolved for the purpose of competition and practise, and the emphasis is on striking correctly rather than hard. Technique and discipline are essential as only the head, torso and hands are targets. Whilst the feet are in motion, the Kendo artist must perform either quick thrusting jabs or high arching blows to reach areas. The strange and intimidating protective armour makes Kendo an extremely impressive and recognisable fighting style.

British Kendo Association

Chapel House
19 Chapel Place
Ramsagte
Kent CT11 9RY
Tel: 020 7515 8653
Website: www.users.dircon.co.uk

All United States Kendo Federation

Website: www.kendo-usa.org

Australian Kendo Renmai

Website: www.akr.aust.com

KICKBOXING

The origins of Full Contact Kick-boxing can be found in Thailand in the 2000 year old discipline of Muay Thai fighting. Thai boxing – like many other martial arts was devised, initially, for self-defence. It only developed into a sport when unarmed combat in warfare became less and less effective. It remains the national sport of Thailand. Thai boxers are awarded the same superstar status in their home nation as premier league footballers in Europe or basketball players in the USA. Full Contact Kick-boxing developed through a combination of Muay Thai and other martial art influences. It was aided in its rise, as were all martial arts at the time, when Bruce Lee exploded onto the big screen.

UK

The Fitness Kickboxing Organization

PO Box 31
Ripley
Derbyshire DE5 8ZX
Tel: 01773 749252

WORLDWIDE

International Kickboxing Federation. World Headquarters in Newcastle, California, USA.
Website: www.ikfkickboxing.com

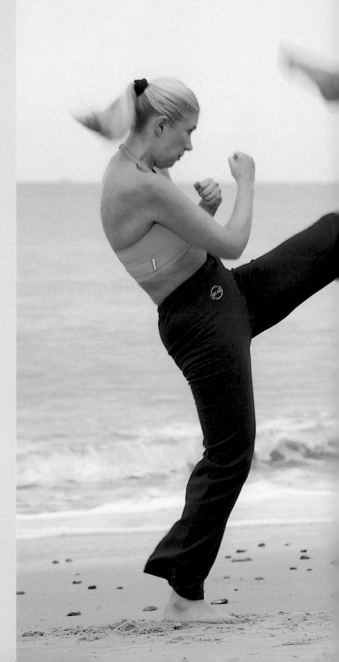

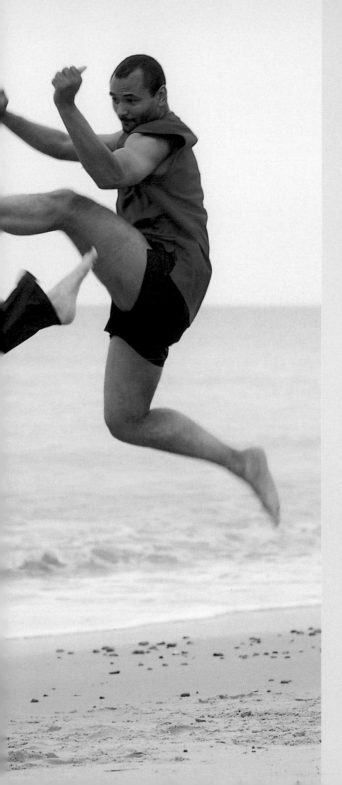

KUNG FU

The style we know today as Kung Fu is the culmination of centuries of many hundreds of styles of Chinese boxing and incorporates philosophies of Daoism and Zen Buddhism. The movement and styles of Kung fu are based on five sacred creatures: crane, dragon, snake, tiger and leopard. Each of these styles has specific stances and actions. One of the best-known styles, popularised in the West by Bruce Lee, is Wing Chun 'beautiful springtime'. This style was developed by a woman and depends largely on speed and momentum – using the hands and feet at close quarters – rather than on brute force. From this style, Bruce Lee further developed his own system, known as Jeet Kune Do 'the way of the intercepting fist'. Many other styles of Kung fu exist, Tai Chi, Hsing I, Paqua, Ti Tang, Tan Tui, Liang I, Tang Lang and Hung Ga.

UK
British Kung Fu Association

Official association for Lua Gar Kung Fu, the best-known style of kung fu.
E-mail: www.laugar-kungfu.co.uk

USA

Website: microbiol.org/vl.martial.martial.arts

AUSTRALIA
Australian School of Kung Fu and Tai Chi

Based in Brisbane, Queensland
Tel: (07) 3869 0484
Website:
www.netspace.net.au/~pagordon/kungfu.htm

MUAY THAI BOXING

Much influenced by Western-style boxing, Muay Thai includes powerful and aggressive kicking techniques, as well as blows with knees and elbows. It can be studied as an effective means of self-defence and in professional competition as a full-contact sport.

Many styles of kick-boxing have developed in the West since Muay Thai was introduced, as it is an adaptable form, able to incorporate techniques from other systems. Modern style kickboxing does not always incorporate knees and elbows to ensure the safety of practitioners.

UK AND WORLDWIDE

Muay Thai Boxing, classes around Epsom and Carshalton, but links countrywide.
Tel: 0956 504068
E-mail: www.scorpions-thai.freeserve.co.uk

USA

Thai Boxing Association of America – the oldest and largest Muay Thai boxing organization in the States founded in 1968 with representatives in most States.
Website: www.thaiboxing.com

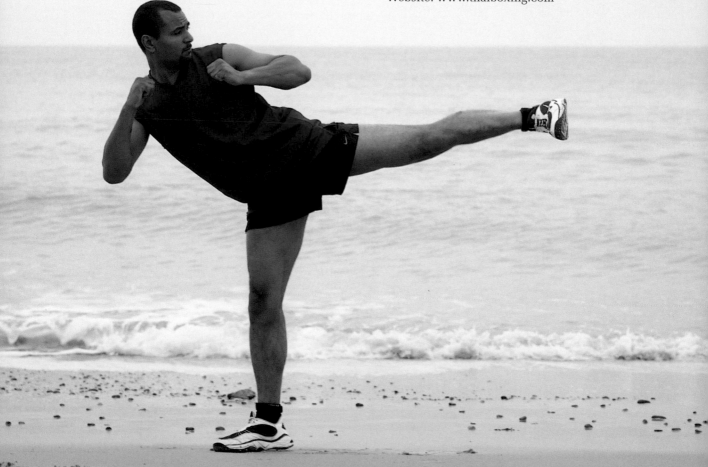

TAE KWON DO

The national martial art of Korea, Tae kwon Do has many similarities and owes much, to the martial arts of its neighbouring countries China and Japan. Kung fu, Karate, Ju-jitsu and Judo have all lent elements to this exciting style. Open-handed combat techniques were extremely important in Korea, so much so that a native art of swordsmanship did not develop.

As well as kicking and punching, jumps, blocks and throws were also used. The modern sport tends to emphasise the legs and kicking techniques, with demanding training and stretching.

Tae kwon do is possibly the most popular martial art practised today in the United States.

UK
British Tae kwon do Council

163a Church Road
Redfield
Bristol BS5 9LA
Tel: 0117 955 1046

Respected dojo run by Martin Ace, a 4th degree black belt Master Instructor.

The Martin Ace Black Belt Academy
77 Chichester Road
Edmonton
London N9 9DH
Tel: 020 8345 5128
Website: www.aceman.co.uk
E-mail tkd@aceman.co.uk

USA
The National Jung Do Kwan Association

Kwanjangnim Frank Clay
Jwan Do Kwan US representative
PO Box 2064 Mechanicsville
VA 23116, USA
Tel: 804 266 5900
Website: americandragon@jungdokwan.net

AUSTRALIA

Melbourne Tae kwon do centre:
www.taekwondo.com.au has links throughout the country.

TAI CHI

This style of martial art has become more familiar as people seek a relaxing, spiritual and healthy exercise to cope with modern stresses. Tai Chi is classed as a 'soft' or 'internal' style of Kung fu, and although benign and peaceful in appearance, is as effective as any hard style in self-defence in application.

Performed in a state of deep relaxation of the body and meditation of the mind, Tai Chi involves constantly flowing circular motions of the arms, legs, hands and feet. These slow, calm movements are carefully balanced, exact and follow set sequences which can take many months to perfect. Ultimately, the goal is to perform the exercises as a constant uninterrupted flow of motion, guided by Chi.

The physical benefits of Tai Chi are numerous, as stamina, flexibility and strength improve. Psychologically, Tai Chi also promotes wellbeing through relaxation and meditation. Unsurprisingly, Tai Chi has deep philosophical roots and applies the theories of cosmic energy, Yin & Yang, and balance in all things.

UK AND USA

Chinese Internal Martial Arts
PO Box 406 Berkeley
California, USA
Tel: 94 701-04 06

AUSTRALIA

Australian Tai Chi Association
PO Box 167 Torrens Park
SA, Australia, 5062
Tel: 041 433 8167
Website: www.sports.org.au/taichi/